Gastric Sleeve Cookbook

Useful Tips to Enjoy Your Favourite Foods After Gastric Sleeve Surgery

(The Comprehensive Guide With Simple and Nourishing Recipes)

Kara Elliott

Published by Sharon Lohan

© **Kara Elliott**

All Rights Reserved

ISBN 978-1-990334-85-6

Legal & Disclaimer

The information contained in this book is not designed to replace or take the place of any form of medicine or professional medical advice. The information in this book has been provided for educational and entertainment purposes only.

Table of contents

Part 1

Introduction To The Digestive System

This system consists of the stomach tract plus the accessory body organs of digestion (the tongue, salivary glands, pancreatic, liver, and gallbladder). Food digestion includes the breakdown of food into smaller as well as smaller sized elements, up until they can be taken in as well as assimilated right into the body. The procedure of food digestion has three stages. The first is the cephalic phase of food digestion, which starts with gastric secretions in feedback to the sight and also the smell of food. This phase consists of the mechanical breakdown of food by eating, and the chemical breakdown by gastrointestinal enzymes, that takes place in the mouth.

Saliva consists of digestive enzymes called amylase, and linguistic lipase, produced by the salivary glands and serous glands on the tongue. The enzymes begin to break down the food in the mouth. Eating, in which the food is blended with saliva, starts the mechanical process of digestion. This creates a bolus that can be ingested down the esophagus to enter the stomach. In the tummy, the gastric phase of food digestion happens. The food is additionally broken down by combining with gastric acid up until it enters the duodenum, in the 3rd digestive phase of food digestion, where it is mixed with many enzymes created by the pancreas. Food digestion is aided by the eating of food accomplished by the muscular tissues of chewing, the tongue, and the teeth, as well as additionally by the tightenings of peristalsis, as well as segmentation. Stomach acid, and the production of mucus in the stomach, are essential for the continuation of food digestion.

Peristalsis is the balanced contraction of muscular tissues that starts in the esophagus as well as continues along the wall surface of the stomach et cetera of the stomach tract. This initially causes the manufacturing of chyme, which, when wholly broken down in the small intestine, is taken in as chyle right into the lymphatic system. Water, as well as some minerals, are reabsorbed back into the blood in the colon of the large intestinal tract. The waste products of food digestion (feces) are excreted from the anus using the rectum.

Components Of The Digestive System

There are several body organs and also other elements associated with the digestion of food. The body organs called the accessory digestion organs are the liver, gall bladder, and even pancreas. Various other components consist of the mouth, salivary glands, tongue, teeth, and epiglottis. The most substantial framework of the gastrointestinal system is the stomach system. This starts at the mouth and also ends at the anus, covering a range of about 9 meters. The most significant part of the GI tract is the colon or large intestine. Water is absorbed below, and also the staying waste matter is saved before defecation.

A lot of the digestion of food happens in the small intestine, which is the longest part of the GI tract. A significant digestive organ is a stomach. Within its mucosa are countless embedded stomach glands. Their secretions are vital to the performance of the body organ. There are several specialist cells in the GI tract. These include the different compartments of the stomach glands, taste cells, pancreatic duct cells, enterocytes, and microfold cells. Some parts of the gastrointestinal system are likewise part of the purgative system, including the vast intestinal tract.

Mouth

It is the first part of the top intestinal tract and also is outfitted with several structures that begin the very first procedures of digestion. These consist of salivary glands, teeth, and even the tongue. The mouth contains two areas; the vestibule and the mouth appropriate. The lobby is the area in between the teeth, lips as well as cheeks, et cetera is the oral cavity proper. A lot of the mouth is lined with dental mucosa, a mucous membrane layer that generates a lubricating mucous, of which just a percentage is required. Mucous membrane layers differ in structure in the various areas of the body. Yet, they all generate a lubricating mucous, which is either produced by surface cells or even more generally by underlying glands. The mucous membrane layer in the mouth proceeds as the thin mucosa, which lines the bases of the teeth. The primary element of mucous is a glycoprotein called mucin, and the type secreted differs according to the region entailed. Mucin is thick, clear, and also clinging.

The roofing of the mouth has described the palate, and also it separates the mouth from the nasal cavity. The taste is hard at the front of the mouth because the overlying mucosa is covering a plate of bone; it is softer as well as extra flexible at the back being made of muscular tissue as well as connective cells, and it can move to ingest food and also fluids. The soft taste buds end at the uvula. The surface area of the problematic taste permits the stress required in consuming food, to leave the nasal passage clear. The opening between the lips is the oral crevice, as well as the opening right into the throat is called the fauces.

At each side of the soft palate are the palatoglossus muscles, which likewise reach into regions of the tongue. These muscle mass raise the rear of the language and additionally close both sides of the fauces to enable food to be ingested. Mucous helps in the chewing of food in its capacity to soften and also collect the food in the development of the bolus.

Salivary glands.

There are three pairs of primary salivary glands and in between 800 as well as 1,000 small salivary glands, all of which generally serve the digestive procedure, and also play an essential role in the upkeep of oral wellness and even general mouth lubrication, without which speech would be impossible. The primary glands are all exocrine glands, secreting via air ducts. The next set is beneath the jaw, the submandibular glands; these produce both serous liquid as well as mucus. Serous glands produce the serous fluid in these salivary glands, which also generate linguistic lipase. They provide regarding 70% of the mouth saliva. The 3rd pair is the sublingual glands located beneath the tongue, and even their secretion is primarily mucous with a small portion of saliva.

The glands likewise produce amylase, an initial stage in the malfunction of food acting upon the carbohydrate in the diet to change the starch material into maltose. There are other severe glands externally of the tongue that encloses taste buds on the back part of the language, and these additionally produce linguistic lipase. Lipase is a gastrointestinal enzyme that catalyzes the hydrolysis of lipids (fats). These glands are termed Von Ebner's organs, which have additionally been revealed to have an additional feature in the secretion of statins, which use very early protection (outside of the immune system) versus germs in food when it reaches these glands on the tongue tissue. Sensory information can stimulate the saliva, supplying the necessary liquid for the tongue to collaborate with as well as likewise to reduce ingesting of the food.

Saliva

Saliva moistens and also softens food, and also, along with the eating action of the teeth, changes the menu right into a smooth bolus. The bolus is then helped by the lubrication supplied by the saliva in its flow from the mouth directly into the esophagus. Also of significance is the visibility in the saliva of the digestive system enzymes amylase and lipase. Saliva is the mouth that can represent 30% of this first starch digestion. Lipase starts to work with breaking down fats. Lipase is even more created in the pancreatic, where it is launched to continue this digestion of fats. The visibility of salivary lipase is of prime significance in young infants whose pancreatic lipase has yet to be developed.

In addition to its duty in supplying digestive system enzymes, saliva has a cleaning activity for the teeth as well as mouth. It additionally has an immunological function in providing antibodies to the system, such as immunoglobulin A.This is attended be type in avoiding infections of the salivary glands, notably that of parotitis.

Saliva also consists of a glycoprotein called haptocorrin, which is a binding protein to vitamin B12. It binds with the vitamin to carry it securely with the acidic content of the stomach. When it gets to the duodenum, pancreatic enzymes break down the glycoprotein and also totally free the vitamin, which after that, binds with the intrinsic aspect.

Tongue

Food enters the mouth where the initial stage in the digestive system procedure takes place, with the action of the language and also the secretion of saliva. The language is a fleshy as well as a muscular sensory body organ, as well as the extremely initial sensory info, is gotten via the palate in the papillae on its surface area. If the taste is good, the tongue will undoubtedly go into activity, controlling the food in the mouth, which promotes the secretion of saliva from the salivary glands. The high fluid quality of the saliva will assist in the conditioning of the food, and also its enzyme content will begin to break down the food while it is in the mouth.

The tongue is linked to the floor of the mouth and also this gives it excellent flexibility for the adjustment of food (and speech); the range of manipulation is optimally controlled by the activity of many muscles and restricted in its external array by the stretch of the frenum. The tongue's two collections of muscles are four intrinsic muscle mass that comes from the tongue. They are included with its shaping, and also four external muscular tissues originating in the bone that is included with its motion.

Taste

Preference is a form of chemoreception that occurs in the specific taste receptors, included in frameworks called palate in the mouth. The palate is mainly on the top surface area (dorsum) of the tongue. The function of preference assumption is essential to aid in preventing damaging or rotten foods from being consumed. There are additionally palate on the epiglottis and top part of the esophagus. The palate is innervated by a branch of the facial nerve, the chorda tympani, and also the glossopharyngeal nerve. Preference messages are sent using these cranial nerves to the mind. The brain can compare the chemical qualities of the food... The discovery of saltiness and also sourness makes it possible for the control of salt as well as acid balance.

The discovery of anger warns of poisons-- most of a plant's supports are of harmful compounds that are bitter. Sweet taste guides to those foods that will supply energy; the first malfunction of the energy-giving carbohydrates by salivary amylase produces the taste of sweet taste because simple sugars are the primary outcome. The preference of umami is thought to signify protein-rich food. Sour flavors are acidic, which is frequently located in lousy food. The mind needs to decide extremely promptly whether the food should be consumed or otherwise. It was the findings in 1991, defining the very first olfactory receptors that helped to prompt the study right into the taste. The olfactory receptors lie on cell surfaces in the nose, which bind to chemicals enabling the discovery of smells. It is presumed that signals from preference receptors work together with those from the nose, to form a suggestion of intricate food flavors.

Teeth

Teeth are complicated frameworks made of materials details to them. They are constructed from a bone-like product called dentin, which is covered by the hardest tissue in the body-- enamel. Teeth have various shapes to deal with different elements of mastication employed in tearing as well as eating items of food into smaller as well as smaller items. This causes a much bigger surface for the action of gastrointestinal enzymes. The teeth are called after their specific functions in the process of chewing-- incisors are utilized for cutting or biting off items of food; canines are used for tearing, premolars, and molars are used for eating and grinding. Chewing of the food with the help of saliva and also mucous results in a soft bolus formation, which can then be ingested to make its means down the upper gastrointestinal system to the stomach. The digestive enzymes in saliva also aid in keeping the teeth clean by breaking down any kind of trapped food fragments.

Epiglottis

It is a flap of elastic cartilage attached to the entryway of the larynx. It is covered with a mucous membrane as well as there is palate on its linguistic surface, which faces into the mouth. Its laryngeal surface encounters into the throat. The epiglottis functions to guard the entry of the glottis, the opening between the singing folds up. It is generally sharp up throughout breathing, with its bottom working as part of the throat. Still, throughout ingesting, the epiglottis folds to an extra horizontal setting, with its upper side operating as part of the pharynx. In this fashion, it avoids food from going into the throat and instead routes it to the esophagus, which lags. Throughout ingesting, the backward movement of the tongue requires the epiglottis over the glottis' opening to protect against any type of food that is being ingested from going into the larynx, which brings about the lungs; the throat is likewise drawn upwards to assist this procedure. Stimulation of the throat by ingested matter creates a strong cough reflex to protect the lungs.

Pharynx

The pharynx belongs to the conducting zone of the respiratory system as well as also a part of the digestive system. It is the part of the throat right away behind the nasal cavity at the rear of the mouth as well as over the esophagus and also larynx. The pharynx is composed of three components. The reduced two parts-- the oropharynx and the laryngopharynx are involved in the gastrointestinal system. The laryngopharynx attaches to the esophagus, and it serves as a passageway for both air and food. Air goes into the throat anteriorly; however, anything swallowed has a concern as well as the flow of air is momentarily blocked. 1465 Muscles in the vocal cords push the food right into the esophagus. The vocal cords join the throat at the oesophageal inlet, which is located behind the cricoid cartilage material.

Esophagus

The esophagus, generally called the food pipe or gullet, consists of a muscular tube where food passes from the vocal cords to the tummy. The throat is constant with the laryngopharynx. It passes the thorax as well as gets in the belly with a hole in the thoracic diaphragm-- the esophageal hiatus, at the level of the tenth thoracic vertebra. Its size averages 25 centimeters, differing with a person's height. It is separated into cervical, thoracic, and abdominal parts. The pharynx signs up with the esophagus at the esophageal inlet, which lags the cricoid cartilage.

At rest, the esophagus is shut at both ends by the top as well as reduced esophageal sphincters. The ingesting response activates the opening of the top sphincter so that food is allowed via. The sphincter additionally offers to stop back circulation from the esophagus into the pharynx. The throat has a mucous membrane, and also the epithelium, which has a safety feature, is continuously replaced as a result of the quantity of food that passes inside the esophagus. Throughout ingesting, food passes from the mouth through the pharynx into the esophagus. The epiglottis folds to a more straight setting to guide the food into the throat, and away from the trachea.

Once in the esophagus, the bolus travels to the tummy through rhythmic tightening as well as relaxation of muscles called peristalsis. The reduced esophageal sphincter is a muscular sphincter surrounding the reduced part of the esophagus. The gastroesophageal junction between the throat as well as the tummy is controlled by the reduced esophageal sphincter, which continues to be constricted at all times, aside from during swallowing and also throwing up to avoid the contents of the belly from going into the esophagus. As the throat does not have the same security from acid as the belly, any failure of this sphincter can result in heartburn.

Diaphragm

The diaphragm is an integral part of the body's gastrointestinal system. The muscle diaphragm separates the thoracic dental caries from the abdominal cavity, where most of the digestive system organs lie. The suspensory muscular tissue connects the ascending duodenum to the diaphragm. This muscle is thought to be helpful in the gastrointestinal system because its add-on uses a more significant angle to the duodenojejunal flexure for the more natural flow of absorbing material. The diaphragm additionally connects to and anchors the liver at its bare area. The esophagus gets in the abdominal region via a hole in the membrane at the level of T10.

The advancement of the gastrointestinal system worries the epithelium of the digestive system and the parenchyma of its derivatives, which originate from the endoderm. Connective cells, muscular parts, as well as peritoneal elements come from the mesoderm. Various regions of the intestine tube such as the esophagus, stomach, duodenum, etc. are specified by a retinoic acid gradient that creates transcription variables one-of-a-kind per area to be expressed. Differentiation of the gut and its by-products depends upon reciprocatory communications between the digestive tract endoderm and its surrounding mesoderm. Hox genes in the mesoderm are induced by a Hedgehog signaling pathway produced by the digestive tract endoderm and regulate the craniocaudal organization of the intestine and also its derivatives. The gut system prolongs from the oropharyngeal membrane layer to the cloacal membrane layer and is split into the foregut, midgut, and also hindgut.

Gastrointestinal Diseases

Food poisonings are the term utilized to refer to any problem or condition that happens within the digestive tract. The stomach system (also called the GI tract) is a collection of hollow organs that create a long passage from our mouth to our anus. The body organs that make up our GI system are our mouth, esophagus, tummy, small intestine, big intestine, as well as anus.

Our GI tract, along with our liver, pancreas, as well as gallbladder, comprise our digestive system. A substantial network of capillary supply blood to these organs and additionally transport nutrients away to other organs in the body. Nerves and hormones collaborate to manage the functioning of the digestive system, and microorganisms that stay within our GI tract (called our gut plants or microbiome) play a role in food digestion, resistance, and also our total health and wellness. A filmy sac called the abdominal muscle holds all the gastrointestinal system organs in position.

Many different conditions or diseases can impact the GI tract as well as have an impact on digestion or our overall health and wellness. Some states have comparable signs, and also additional medical investigations may be required before a physician gets to a diagnosis. Common gastrointestinal disorders include:

Gastric disease: Gastric illness is a significant autoimmune problem where the small intestine is oversensitive to gluten. Intake of gluten creates the body's immune system of the body to assault the small intestine, resulting in damage to the villi of the small intestine, which are little fingerlike estimates that advertise nutrition absorption.

The gastric disease can begin at any type of age, as well as signs and symptoms include bloating, modifications in digestive tract routine (either looseness of the bowels or irregular bowel movements), breakouts, weight loss, as well as a low growth price in youngsters. Presently, the only therapy for gastric disease is lifelong adherence to a rigorous gluten-free diet regimen.

Bowel irregularity: Constipation is the term made use of to define trouble or infrequency in passing stools (feces). Not everyone has a daily bowel movement, so the passage of time between bowel movements before bowel irregularity occurs differs from person to person. When someone is constipated, their feces are generally tiny, robust, dehydrated, and tough to pass. Various other signs might consist of bloating or distention in the belly and discomfort throughout defecation. Hemorrhoids frequently accompany constipation. There are multiple sources of irregular bowel movements, such as dehydration, a lack of fiber in the diet, maternity, inactivity, or specific drugs (such as antidepressants, iron supplements, or opioids). Laxatives can assist relieve irregularity, and also a way of life changes can help stop it from repeating.

Crohn's Disease: It is a digestive tract disease that causes patches of swelling in the GI tract between the mouth and also the rectum. However, the location where the small intestine joins the enormous intestinal tract is most typically affected. The specific reason continues to be unknown; nonetheless, it is extra usual in "Westernized" nations, tends to run in households, and also diet regimen and stress and anxiety might worsen the illness.

Signs might consist of diarrhea that continues for many weeks, stomach discomfort, and also weight loss. Around 50% of individuals with Crohn's illness notice blood or mucous in their feces as well as some may report an urgent requirement to relocate their bowels or experience of incomplete discharge. Medicine treatments may consist of aminosalicylates, corticosteroids, immunomodulators, as well as biologics. Surgical procedures might likewise be an alternative.

Diarrhea: Signs of diarrhea consist of constant, loosened, watery feces (feces), which are usually accompanied by an immediate demand to visit the toilet. Abdominal pain or cramping may additionally occur, and also in some cases queasiness or vomiting. Infections are a usual reason for diarrhea, particularly noroviruses, which are the usual cause of diarrhea and vomiting outbreaks on cruise ships. Other typical reasons include microorganisms, such as salmonella, campylobacter, or Escherichia coli giardia; some clinical issues (such as a Celiac condition or Crohn's illness); food intolerance or medications. Anti-diarrhea medicines such as loperamide or diphenoxylate help slow down bowel movements, and also electrolyte options are beneficial for dealing with dehydration, which frequently accompanies excessive looseness of the bowels. In some cases, other medications, such as antibiotics, may likewise be required.

Diverticular condition: Diverticular disease is a persistent condition in which tiny pockets or outpouchings, called diverticula, happen in the bowel. Diverticula can come to be irritated when undigested food gets entrapped within them, causing discomfort and irregular bowel movements, and often fever, queasiness, or cramping. This is called diverticulitis. Diverticular disease is common, influencing half of all individuals over 60. A reduced fiber diet is thought to be the main reason, although some individuals have a genetic proneness to the illness. Lots of people with diverticular disease do not have signs and symptoms, as well as the problem is usually uncovered during a colonoscopy to screen for intestines cancer cells. Therapy is generally with a high-fiber diet as well as a mild pain reliever.

Gastroesophageal Reflux Illness (GERD): GERD is likewise called heartburn or indigestion. It takes place when the ring of muscle fibers that borders the entryway to our belly (called the reduced esophageal sphincter) comes to be weak, and also rather than staying securely near to avoid the backflow of food back up our esophagus, it remains partially open, enabling partially digested food as well as belly acid to leak back up the esophagus, irritating. The first signs and symptoms connected with GERD are regurgitation, heartburn, breast discomfort, and also queasiness. GERD is most typically treated with antacids, H2 blockers, or Proton Pump Inhibitors.

Piles as well as anal crevices: Piles take place when the rectal cushions (which are little areas of vein-containing cells that secure the rectal opening, stopping urinary incontinence) come to be engorged as well as swollen. They can occur externally or internally, and both types commonly hemorrhage when a bowel movement is passed. Outside piles look like little bunches of grapes and can end up being really red, tender, and also itchy when irritated. Internal piles can trigger a feeling of stress inside the rectum and also are generally not visible. Sometimes they may prolapse ("pop") out of the rectum complying with a digestive tract activity, which can be quite unpleasant. Therapy is with hemorrhoid creams or suppositories. Other specialized treatments, such as sclerotherapy, laser therapy, or surgery might be required.

Rectal fissures are little tears in the slim tissue that lines the anus. They are common in infants and also commonly happen when passing substantial bowel movements. Laxatives and also a high fiber diet plan can make it simpler to pass feces and also stop anal fissures from developing.

Irritable Bowel Syndrome (IBS): the American College of Gastroenterology defines IBS as "Stomach discomfort related to modified digestive tract behaviors." It generally takes most individuals three years and at the very least three different doctors before they are given a diagnosis of IBS. Part of the problem with medical diagnosis rests with the many different presentations of IBS. Some individuals are most likely to have irregular bowel movements (constipation-predominant IBS or IBS-C), others diarrhea (diarrhea-predominant IBS or IBS-D), while a couple of experience both bowel irregularity and also diarrhea at different times (blended IBS). Signs and symptoms are additionally comparable to numerous various other conditions, such as endometriosis, giardia, food allergies, or inflammatory digestive tract condition, as well as most of these problems that need to be left out before a medical diagnosis of IBS can be made. Treatment relies on what type of IBS a person has (i.e., either irregular bowel movements or looseness of the bowels primary) and consists typically of medicine and also dietary changes.

Lactose intolerance: People with it do not generate adequate of the enzyme lactase, and find it difficult to digest lactose. It is more usual in people of Asian, Center Eastern, Mediterranean, South American, or African descent, as well as can additionally be brought on by gut damage (such as that following gastroenteritis or surgical treatment) or with conditions such as Celiac or Crohn's disease. Signs and symptoms usually consist of wind, bloating, stomach discomfort, nausea, or diarrhea within thirty minutes to 2 hrs after consuming something with lactose.

Malabsorption disorders: Malabsorption disorders refer to a variety of different problems in which the small intestine is incapable of taking in nutrients, such as healthy proteins, carbs, fats, vitamins, or minerals. There are numerous root causes of malabsorption syndrome, such as prolonged use of prescription antibiotics, illness of the gallbladder, liver, or pancreatic, problems such as Crohn's condition, gastric condition, persistent pancreatitis, and cystic fibrosis, and congenital disabilities. Treatment depends upon the underlying problem and also the degree of malabsorption.

Polyps and intestines cancer cells: Polyps are growths that happen on the internal surface of the colon. There are two primary kinds. One type (adenomas or adenomatous polyps) have a high threat of turning into colorectal cancer as well as should be removed if located.

Colon cancer is the third source of cancer cells deaths amongst American males and females. Many colorectal cancer cells grow slowly and also trigger a couple of signs until they reach a large size, which is why colon cancer cell testing is so essential since colorectal cancer cells are more common in individuals aged 45 with to 75 years. Therapy of colon cancer relies on which stage the cancer cells are located and also might consist of surgical treatment, radiation treatment, and even radiation therapy.

Peptic Ulcer Condition (PUD): Peptic ulcer disease is an umbrella term used to define both stomach and also duodenal abscess, which are tiny holes that can occur in the lining of your stomach (stomach ulcer) or upper part of your small intestine (duodenal ulcers). Duodenal ulcers are one of the most typical kind as well as are more probable in men aged between 30 as well as half a century. Stomach abscess frequently affects middle-aged or senior people.

The most usual cause is an infection with a germ called Helicobacter pylori (H. pylori), which is typically gotten in childhood, although the majority of people never establish abscess. Overuse of anti-inflammatory drugs such as pain killers, Advil, or diclofenac, too much acid production in the belly, and smoking cigarettes are additionally usual causes. Symptoms typically include abdominal pain and also heartburn. The pain of duodenal ulcers tends to be eased by food, whereas the pain with gastric ulcers is worsened by consuming. Therapy usually consists of drugs to decrease acid manufacturing in the stomach or to shield the tummy, and treatment to eradicate H. pylori infection.

Ulcerative colitis: Ulcerative colitis affects just the innermost lining of the colon. Although the colon is the only part of the digestive tract impacted, the whole of the colon is inflamed. Signs and symptoms resemble Crohn's illness and consist of diarrhea, as well as the frequent demand to have defecation (additionally called tenesmus). Pus, as well as mucus, might also happen as a result of abscess that creates in the colon. Other symptoms include anal blood loss or bloody feces, stomach discomfort, exhaustion, and loss of appetite. The reason continues to be unknown, although an uncommon immune response appears responsible for the swelling, and also diet, as well as anxiety, exacerbate the condition. Genetics also seems to play a role. Treatment is with corticosteroids, antidiarrheal agents, immunomodulators as well as biologics, depending on disease seriousness.

Vomiting: Vomiting is when the components of the stomach are powerfully gotten rid of via the mouth, generally unwillingly. Nausea is the term utilized to describe sensation sick-- or like you are practically to vomit. Infection from bacteria, viruses, or other microorganisms is one of the most usual sources of throwing up. Overindulgence in alcohol, food allergies, migraine headaches, and also pregnancy might likewise create vomiting. Therapy depends on the reason and also may include antiemetics and rehydration services, depending on exactly how suitable these are for the individual with the vomiting.

What Is The Stomach?

The stomach is a muscular organ in the intestinal tract of humans and many other pets, consisting of several invertebrates. The tummy has a dilated framework and operates as a crucial digestive system body organ. In the gastrointestinal system, the belly is involved in the 2nd stage of digestion, adhering to eating. It carries out a chemical failure as a result of enzymes and hydrochloric acid.

In people and also lots of other pets, the stomach is located in between the gullet as well as the small intestine. It secretes digestive enzymes and also gastric acid to aid in food digestion. The pyloric sphincter regulates the passage of partially absorbed food (chyme) from the tummy right into the duodenum, where peristalsis takes control of to move this via the rest of the intestines.

The stomach is a significant body organ of the stomach system and also the gastrointestinal system. It is a continually J-shaped body organ signed up with to the esophagus at its top end and the duodenum at its reduced end. Stomach acid (informally stomach juice), generated in the stomach plays a vital role in the digestion procedure, and mainly includes hydrochloric acid and also sodium chloride. A peptide hormonal agent, gastrin, created by G cells in the gastric glands, boosts the production of gastric juice, which turns on the digestion enzymes. Pepsinogen is a forerunner enzyme (zymogen) generated by the gastric chief cells, as well as stomach acid triggers this to the enzyme pepsin, which starts the digestion of proteins. As these two chemicals would harm the tummy wall, mucous is produced by many gastric glands in the tummy, to provide a slimed safety layer against the harmful results of the chemicals on the internal sheets of the belly.

At the same time that healthy protein is being digested, mechanical churning takes place with the activity of peristalsis, waves of muscular contractions that move along the belly wall. This permits the mass of food to more blend with the digestion enzymes. Gastric lipase produced by the chief cells in the fundic glands in the stomach mucosa of the tummy, is an acidic lipase, in contrast with the alkaline pancreatic lipase. This breaks down fats to some extent though it is not as efficient as the pancreatic lipase.

The pylorus, which attaches to the duodenum via the pyloric canal, includes many glands that produce gastrointestinal enzymes, including gastrin. After an hr or 2, a thick semi-liquid called chyme is created. When the pyloric sphincter or shutoff opens up, chyme gets in the duodenum where it mixes better with digestion enzymes from the pancreas, and after that passes through the small intestine, where digestion proceeds.

When the chyme is completely digested, it is soaked up right into the blood. 95% of the absorption of nutrients takes place in the small intestine. Water and minerals are absorbed back into the blood in the colon of the vast intestinal tract, where the environment is slightly acidic. Some vitamins, such as biotin as well as vitamin K produced by germs in the gut of the colon are also absorbed.

The parietal cells in the tummy, generate a glycoprotein called a natural element, which is essential for vitamin B12. Vitamin B12 is carried to, as well as with the tummy, bound to a glycoprotein secreted by the salivary glands - transcobalamin I, likewise called haptocorrin, which secures the acid-sensitive vitamin from the acidic stomach components. As soon as in the extra neutral duodenum, pancreatic enzymes break down the safety glycoprotein. The freed vitamin B12 then binds to the innate aspect, which is then absorbed by the enterocytes in the ileum.

The stomach is a distensible body organ and can generally increase to hold concerning one liter of food. This growth is allowed by a collection of gastric folds up in the inner walls of the tummy. The tummy of a newborn baby will just be able to increase to preserve regarding 30 ml.

Stomach Conditions

Gastroesophageal reflux: Stomach components, consisting of acid, can take a trip backward up the esophagus. There may be no symptoms, or reflux might cause heartburn or coughing.

Gastroesophageal reflux condition (GERD): When signs of reflux become bothersome or happen frequently, they're called GERD. Infrequently, GERD can cause significant issues of the esophagus.

Dyspepsia: Another name for indigestion or acid indigestion. Dyspepsia may be brought on by practically any benign or severe condition that impacts the tummy.

Gastric ulcer (belly ulcer): An erosion in the cellular lining of the stomach, commonly triggering pain and bleeding. Stomach ulcers are frequently triggered by NSAIDs or H. pylori infection.

Peptic ulcer illness: Physicians consider abscess in either the belly or the duodenum (the first part of the small intestine) peptic ulcer condition.

Gastritis: Swelling of the belly, often creating queasiness and pain. Gastritis can be brought on by alcohol, specific medicines, H. pylori infection, or other factors.

Belly cancer cells: Gastric cancer is an uncommon kind of cancer cells in the U.S. Adenocarcinoma, and also lymphoma comprises a lot of the situations of tummy cancer.

Zollinger-Ellison syndrome (ZES): One or more growths that produce hormonal agents that lead to boosted acid production. Severe GERD, as well as peptic ulcer disease results from this rare disorder.

Stomach varices: In people with severe liver illness, capillaries in the belly might swell and bulge under boosted stress. Called varices, these veins go to danger for bleeding, although less so than esophageal varices are.

Stomach bleeding: Gastritis, abscess, or gastric cancers might hemorrhage. Seeing blood or black product in vomit or feces is generally a medical emergency.

Gastroparesis (postponed gastric draining): Nerve damages from diabetic issues or other problems may harm the stomach's muscle contractions. Queasiness, as well as vomiting, are common signs.

Stomach Test

Upper endoscopy (esophagogastroduodenoscopy or EGD): A flexible tube with an electronic camera on its end (endoscope) is placed through the mouth. The endoscope enables the evaluation of the esophagus, belly, and also duodenum (the first part of the small intestine).

Calculated tomography (CT check): A CT scanner makes use of X-rays and also a computer system to develop images of the stomach as well as abdomen.

Magnetic vibration imaging: Using a magnetic field, a scanner develops high-resolution photos of the tummy and abdomen.

pH testing: Utilizing a tube with the nose into the esophagus, acid levels in the throat can be kept an eye on. This can assist in identifying or change treatment for GERD.

Barium swallow: After swallowing barium, X-ray films of the esophagus and also belly are taken. This can occasionally detect ulcers or various other troubles.

Upper GI collection: X-rays are taken of the esophagus, stomach, and top part of the small intestine.

Gastric emptying study: A test of just how quickly food goes through the tummy. The food is identified with a chemical as well as checked out on a scanner.

Stomach biopsy: During an endoscopy, a physician can take a small item of stomach cells for tests. This can diagnose H. pylori infection, cancer cells, or other problems.

H. pylori examination: While the majority of people with H. pylori infection do not establish ulcers, straightforward blood or feces examinations can be done to check for infection in individuals with ulcers or to validate that the disease is erased after treatment.

Stomach Treatments

Histamine (H2) blockers: Histamine increases tummy acid secretion; blocking histamine can lower acid production as well as GERD signs.

Proton pump preventions: These medications straight hinder the acid pumps in the stomach. They need to be taken daily to be effective.

Antacids: These medications can aid versus the results of acid but don't kill germs or stop acid manufacturing.

Endoscopy: Throughout a top endoscopy, tools on the endoscope can occasionally quit tummy bleeding, if present.

Mobility agents: Medicines can raise contraction of the tummy, enhancing signs of gastroparesis.

Stomach surgical treatment: Cases of extreme stomach blood loss, burst abscess, or cancer need a surgical procedure to be healed.

Anti-biotics: H. pylori infection can be treated with antibiotics, which are taken with other medicines to recover the tummy.

Structure Of Stomach

In people, the tummy exists between the esophagus as well as the duodenum (the very first part of the small intestine). Existing behind the tummy is pancreatic. A substantial double fold of natural peritoneum called the higher omentum suspends from, the better curvature of the stomach. Two sphincters keep the contents of the tummy contained; the lower oesophageal sphincter (found in the cardiac region), at the joint of the esophagus as well as belly, and also the pyloric sphincter at the joint of the stomach with the duodenum.

The tummy is surrounded by parasympathetic (energizer) and sympathetic (prevention) plexuses (networks of capillary and also nerves in the anterior gastric, posterior, exceptional and substandard, gastric and myenteric), which control both the secretory task of the tummy and even the motor (activity) activity of its muscular tissues.

Because it is a distensible body organ, it generally expands to hold about one liter of food. The tummy of a newborn human baby will only be able to retain regarding 30 milliliters. The optimum stomach quantity in adults is between 2 as well as 4 liters.

Sections

The belly has four central anatomical departments; the cardia, fundus, body as well as pylorus:

Cardia-- surrounds the superior opening of the tummy at the T11 level.

Fundus-- the rounded, often gas filled up portion above as well as left of the cardia.

Body-- the sizeable main section inferior to the fundus.

Pylorus-- This location attaches the stomach to the duodenum. It is split right into the pyloric antrum, pyloric canal, and pyloric sphincter. The pyloric sphincter demarcates the transpyloric airplane at the degree of L1.

Anatomical closeness

The tummy bed refers to the structures, after which the belly rests in creatures. These consist of the pancreatic, spleen, left kidney, left suprarenal gland, transverse colon, and also its mesocolon and the diaphragm. The term was presented around 1896 by Philip Polson of the Catholic University School of Medication, Dublin. Nonetheless, this was brought into disrepute by doctor anatomist J Massey.

Blood supply

The minimal curvature of the human belly is supplied by the ideal stomach artery inferiorly as well as the left gastric artery superiorly, which also provides the cardiac region. The better curvature is provided by the appropriate gastroepiploic artery inferiorly and the left gastroepiploic artery superiorly. The fundus of the belly, and additionally the upper portion of the higher curvature, is supplied by the short gastric arteries, which develop from the splenic artery.

Microanatomy

Wall

Like the various other parts of the gastrointestinal tract, the human stomach wall surfaces contain a mucosa, submucosa, muscularis externa, subserosa, and serosa. The internal part of the lining of the stomach, the stomach mucosa, includes an external layer of cells, a lamina propria, and a slim layer of smooth muscle mass called the mucosa. Beneath the mucosa lies the submucosa. Meissner's plexus is in this layer.

Outside of the submucosa exists an additional muscle layer, the muscular externa. It consists of three layers of muscular fibers, with fibers existing at angles per other. These are the internal oblique, inner circular, as well as external longitudinal layers.

The internal oblique layer: This layer is in charge of creating the movement that churns and also breaks down the food. It is the layer of the three, which is not seen in various other parts of the gastrointestinal system. The antrum has skin cells in its walls and also carries out much more strong tightenings than the fundus.

The middle round layer: At this layer, the pylorus is bordered by a thick round muscular wall surface, which is usually tonically tightened, developing a functional (if not anatomically discrete) pyloric sphincter, which regulates the activity of chyme right into the duodenum.

Auerbach's plexus (AKA myenteric plexus) is discovered between the external longitudinal and the center circular layer and is in charge of the innervation of both (creating peristalsis and mixing). The outer longitudinal layer is in the cost of relocating the bolus in the direction of the pylorus of the belly through muscular reduction. To the beyond the muscular externa exists a serosa, including layers of connective cells continual with the abdominal muscle.

GlandsThe mucosa lining the belly is lined with a number of these pits, which receive stomach juice, secreted by between 2 and 7 stomach glands. Stomach juice is an acidic liquid having hydrochloric acid and also the gastrointestinal enzyme pepsin. Within the organs has many cells, with the function of the glands changing, relying on their setting within the belly.

Glands differ where the stomach meets the gorge, and also near the pylorus. Near the junction between the tummy and the esophagus lie cardiac glands, which mostly produce mucous. They are few in number than the other gastric glands and also are extra shallowly positioned in the mucosa. There are two kinds - either basic tubular with short ducts or compound racemose resembling the duodenal Brunner's glands.

Genetics and healthy protein expression.

About 20,000 healthy protein-coding genetics are revealed in human cells, and also almost 70% of these genetics are shown in the regular belly. Just over 150 of these genetics are extra explicitly expressed in the stomach compared to other body organs, with only some 20 genetics being highly detailed. The matching particular healthy proteins expressed in the tummy are mostly involved in creating an appropriate atmosphere for managing the food digestion of food for the uptake of nutrients. Highly stomach-specific proteins include GKN1, revealed in the mucosa; pepsinogen PGC and also the lipase LIPF, expressed in primary cells; and even stomach ATPase ATP4A as well as gastric intrinsic factor GIF, shared in parietal cells.

Functions Of Stomach

The tummy is a bean-shaped sack situated behind the lower ribs. Once food hits the stomach, sphincters of the tummy as well as the leave right into the small intestine close. The lining of the belly then secretes hydrochloric acids and enzymes that break down the food to make sure that it can advance its journey through the gastrointestinal system, according to the Cleveland Facility. As it secretes acid and enzymes, the abdominal muscle agreement in a procedure called peristalsis to blend the food with the enzymes.

The acid likewise works to kill harmful germs that might have made their method right into the body together with food as well as beverage. The acid might damage the tummy, so it secretes a sticky, neutralizing mucus that layers its walls and protects it from damages. The stomach likewise makes a compound that is needed for the body to soak up vitamin B12, according to the Digestion Illness Facility (DDC).

The tummy is the most significant part of the digestive system. It does not just absorb food; it likewise keeps it. According to the BBC, the belly can hold a bit greater than a quart (1 liter) of food simultaneously. The design of the stomach enables an individual to eat a large meal that can be digested slowly gradually. It can take 4 to six hours or longer to absorb a meal, according to the BBC. The higher the fat web content of the food, the longer it considers the food to digest.

Digestion

In the digestive system, a bolus (a small rounded mass of chewed out food) goes into the belly via the esophagus using the reduced esophageal sphincter. The stomach launches proteases (protein-digesting enzymes such as pepsin) and also hydrochloric acid, which kills or prevents microorganisms and also offers an acidic pH of 2 for the proteases to work. The belly spins food with muscular contractions of the wall surface called peristalsis-- minimizing the quantity of the bolus, before looping the fundus as well as the body of a belly as they're converted into chyme (partially digested food).

Chyme slowly goes through the pyloric sphincter and also right into the duodenum of the small intestine, where the removal of nutrients begins. Gastric juice in the stomach likewise has pepsinogen. Hydrochloric acid triggers this inactive type of enzyme into the active type, pepsin. Pepsin breaks down proteins into polypeptides.

Absorption

Although the absorption in the human digestion system is mostly a function of the small intestine, some absorption of specific little molecules, however, does occur in the tummy via its lining. This consists of:

- Water, if the body is dried out

- The drug, such as pain killers

- Amino acids

- 10-- 20% of ingested ethanol

- High levels of caffeine

- To a little level, water-soluble vitamins (most are soaked up in the small intestine).

The parietal cells of the human belly are accountable for creating an inherent element, which is essential for the absorption of vitamin B12. B12 is made use of in the mobile metabolic process and also is needed for the production of red cells, and the performance of the nerve system.

Control of secretion as well as motility.

The motion and also the flow of chemicals right into the tummy are regulated by both the free nerves as well as by the numerous gastrointestinal hormonal agents of the digestive system.

Gastrin.

The hormonal agent gastrin triggers an increase in the secretion of HCl from the parietal cells and pepsinogen from the chief cells in the stomach. It additionally causes raised mobility in the stomach. It is released by G cells in the belly in response to distension of the antrum, as well as digestive system products (specifically vast quantities of incompletely absorbed proteins). It is inhibited by a pH usually less than 4 (high acid), as well as the hormone somatostatin.

Cholecystokinin.

Cholecystokinin (CCK) has the most effect on the gall bladder, triggering gall bladder contractions. Still, it additionally lowers gastric draining as well as boosts the release of pancreatic juice, which is alkaline and also reduces the effects of the chyme—I-cells manufacture CCK in the mucosal epithelium of the small intestine.

Secretin

Differently and uncommonly, secretin, which has most impacts on the pancreas, likewise diminish acid secretion in the belly. Secretin is manufactured by S-cells, which lie in the duodenal mucosa as well as in the jejunal mucosa in smaller numbers.

Gastric repressive peptide.

Gastric inhibitory peptide (GIP) reduces both gastric acid launch as well as mobility. GIP is synthesized by K-cells, which lie in the duodenal and jejunal mucosa.

Enteroglucagon.

Enteroglucagon reduces both gastric acid and also mobility. Besides gastrin, these hormonal agents all act to turn off the belly activity. This remains in reaction to foodstuff in the liver and also gall bladder, which has not yet been taken in. The belly press food right into the small intestine only when the pipe is not busy while the organ is full and still digesting food, the stomach functions as storage space for food.

Results of EGF.

The skin development variable (EGF) results in cellular proliferation, differentiation, and survival. [30] EGF is a low-molecular-weight polypeptide first detoxified from the computer mouse submandibular gland, but ever since located in lots of human cells consisting of the submandibular gland, and also the parotid gland. Salivary EGF, which also appears to be regulated by nutritional inorganic iodine, likewise plays an essential physical duty in the upkeep of oro-oesophageal and stomach cells' integrity. The natural results of salivary EGF include recovery of oral and gastroesophageal ulcers, restraint of stomach acid secretion, the excitement of DNA synthesis, and also mucosal protection from intraluminal damaging variables such as gastric acid, bile acids, pepsin, and also trypsin and also from physical, chemical, and bacterial representatives.

Tummy as a nourishment sensor.

The human belly can "taste" sodium glutamate using glutamate receptors, and also this information is passed to the side hypothalamus and limbic system in the brain as a palatability signal with the vagus nerve. The belly can additionally pick up, independently of the tongue and also oral preference receptors, sugar, carbohydrates, healthy proteins, and even fats. This enables the brain to link dietary worth of foods to their tastes.

Thyrogastric syndrome.

This syndrome defines the association between thyroid condition and also chronic gastritis, which was first described in the 1960s. This term was created additionally to indicate the visibility of thyroid autoantibodies or autoimmune thyroid condition in individuals with destructive anemia, a late medical stage of atrophic gastritis. In 1993, has been published a full examination on the tummy and also thyroid, reporting that the thyroid is, embryo genetically and also phylogenetically, stemmed from the primitive belly, which the thyroid cells, moved and too focused on the uptake of iodide as well as in storage space and explanation of iodine compounds. Stomach and thyroid share iodine capability and several morphological resemblances, such as cell polarity and also apical microvilli, similar organ-specific antigens as well as additionally associated autoimmune diseases, secretion of glycoproteins (thyroglobulin and also mucin) and even peptide hormones, the digesting as well as reabsorbing ability and, finally, the similar capability to create iodotyrosines by peroxidase task, where iodide acts as electron contributor in the presence of H_2O_2. In complying with years, lots of scientists released testimonials concerning this disorder.

Diseases Of Stomach

The stomach is an essential organ in the body. It plays a crucial function in digestion of foods, launches different enzymes as well as additionally protects the lower intestinal tract from unsafe microorganisms. The belly links to the esophagus over as well as to the small intestine listed below. It is elaborately related to the pancreas, spleen, and also liver. The stomach does vary in dimension, yet its J form is constant. The tummy depends on the upper part of the abdominal area just listed below the left chest.

Instances consisting of the name gastropathy include portal hypertensive gastropathy as well as Ménétrier's condition, likewise known as "hyperplastic hypersecretory gastropathy." Nonetheless, many various other stomach illnesses don't include the word "gastropathy" such as gastric or peptic ulcer conditions, gastroparesis, as well as dyspepsia.

Many belly diseases are connected with infection. Historically, it was extensively believed that the highly acidic environment of the tummy would undoubtedly maintain the stomach immune from contagion. However, many studies have indicated that many situations of tummy ulcers, gastritis, as well as stomach cancer are triggered by Helicobacter pylori infection. One of the methods it can make it through in the belly includes its urease enzymes, which metabolize urea (which is generally produced into the stomach) to ammonia as well as co2, which neutralizes gastric acid and also, therefore, stops its food digestion. In recent times, it has been discovered that other Helicobacter germs are even with the ability to colonize the stomach and also have been connected with gastritis.

Having little or no gastric acid is referred to as hypochlorhydria or achlorhydria specifically as well as are conditions that can have adverse wellness influences. Having high levels of stomach acid is called hyperchlorhydria. Many people believe that hyperchlorhydria can cause tummy abscess. Nonetheless, the current research study indicates that the stomach mucosa, which produces stomach acid, is acid-resistant.

Numerous types of persistent conditions impact the stomach. However, given that the signs and symptoms are localized to this organ, the regular symptoms of stomach issues consist of nausea or vomiting, vomiting, bloating, cramps, looseness of the bowels, and discomfort.

The tummy can have several conditions and also an illness that can cause discomfort, discomfort, digestion troubles as well as even death. One of the most common tummy problems is indigestion or dyspepsia. "Dyspepsia is a term used to describe several signs and symptoms, including a sensation of volume throughout a meal, uneasy fullness after a dish, as well as burning or discomfort in the top abdominal area," Dr. Lisa Ganjhu, professional assistant professor of medicine and also a gastroenterologist at NYU Langone Medical Center, told Live Science.

Upper stomach pain, indigestion, and also heartburn affects around 25 percent of the populace each year, according to the DDC. Therapy of upset stomach generally relies on the cause.

GERD occurs when acid contents in the tummy get refluxed up right into the esophagus. Spicy foods, mint, delicious chocolate, caffeine, alcohol, or citrus foods raise swelling or level of acidity in the stomach, which can cause reflux. Foods that take longer to digest can make GERD signs and symptoms even worse. Stress and also anxiousness can likewise add to GERD, claimed Ganjhu.

Belly ulcers are breaks in the cellular lining of the tummy, brought on by certain medications as well as way too much acid in the stomach. These are exposed to the acids in the belly, causing pain. In many cases, ulcers can conveniently be treated with the drug.

Tummy cancer cells are cancer cells that come from the tummy. According to the U.S. (NLM), it mostly affects older people. Two-thirds of the people impacted with stomach cancer more than age 65. In its innovative stages, some signs of stomach cancer are unexplained weight reduction, vomiting, blood in the stool, jaundice, or problem ingesting. Around 10,720 individuals pass away from tummy cancer yearly, according to the American Cancer Culture.

Belly influenza isn't the flu in any way. It is a stomach virus. Flu affects the respiratory system, not the gastrointestinal tract. According to the Mayo Center, some usual signs are watery, generally non-bloody looseness of the bowels, abdominal cramps, vomiting, nausea or vomiting, muscle mass pains, headache, and also low-grade high temperature.

Problems of the belly are typical and also cause a considerable amount of morbidity as well as suffering in the populace. Information from healthcare facilities shows that greater than 25% of the populace suffers from some sort of persistent stomach condition, including abdominal discomfort and also acid indigestion. These signs and symptoms happen for long periods and trigger long term suffering, time off the job as well as low quality of life. Moreover, check outs to physicians, the expense of examinations, and also treatment lead to many days shed from the job and a colossal price to the monetary system.

Cancers cells

Cancers of the stomach are unusual as well as the occurrence has been decreasing worldwide. Stomach cancers batteries regularly happen as a result of variations in the level of acidity level and also may provide unclear signs and symptoms of stomach fullness, weight management as well as discomfort. The actual source of belly cancer is not known yet has been connected to infection with Helicobacter pylori, pernicious anemia, Meniere's disease, and nitrogenous chemicals in food.

Crohn's disease

Crohn's condition is an inflammatory bowel condition that can influence any type of part of the digestion system, even the belly, although it's a rare presentation. Symptoms include abdominal discomfort, anorexia nervosa, and also fat burning. Diarrhea is also a sign that can create, so inspecting stools for the look of blood is essential. It is feasible for symptoms of Crohn's condition to stay with an individual for weeks or vanish by themselves. Coverage the signs to a medical professional is advised to avoid additional difficulties.

Gastroparesis

One more widespread, long-term problem, which is currently a lot more valued is gastroparesis. Gastroparesis influences countless individuals and is usually never believed, and most individuals have a delay in medical diagnosis. Necessarily in gastroparesis, the tummy motility goes away as well as food stays stationary in the stomach. The most common root cause of gastroparesis is diabetes, but it can also happen from a clog at the distal end of the belly, cancer, or a stroke. Signs of gastroparesis include abdominal discomfort, fullness, bloating, nausea, vomiting after eating food, anorexia nervosa, and feeling of fullness after eating percentages of food.

Gastritis

In the belly, there is a small equilibrium between acid and the wall lining, which is safeguarded by mucous. When this mucus cellular lining is interfered with for whatever factor, symptoms, and signs of the level of acidity result. This might lead to top stomach pain, indigestion, anorexia nervosa, nausea, throwing up as well as heartburn. When the problem is allowed to advance, the pain might become continuous; blood may begin to leakage and be seen in the feces. If the blood loss is fast and also of appropriate quantity, it may also cause vomiting of bright red blood (hematemesis). When the level of acidity is unrestrained, it can also cause extreme blood loss (anemia) or lead to opening (hole) in the tummy, which is a medical emergency. In many people, the active bleeding from an abscess blends with the feces as well as offers as black feces. The presence of blood in stools is commonly the initial sign that there is trouble in the belly.

Promoting excellent stomach health

Ganjhu offers these tips for the very best method to prevent gastrointestinal problems such as bowel irregularity and also indigestion:

- Consume little meals.

- Stay clear of all soft drinks.

- Eat a diet plan rich in fruits and vegetables, and minimize fatty foods.

- Quit smoking cigarettes.

- Slim down.

- After meals, take a walk.

- Prevent bedtime snacks.

- Avoid annoying foods.

- Drink eight glasses of water or other non-caffeinated fluid each day.

- Usage acid-blocking drugs, if required.

- Load up on fiber to bulk your feces. Eat at the very least, 25 to 30 grams of fiber daily.

- Workout 30 to 40 minutes, three to 5 times a week, to assist with total stomach (GI) wellness. Strolling, running, weight training/resistance training all assistance.

- Eat probiotics to maintain the microbiome healthy and balanced if you have GI issues.

- Bowel movement when you have the urge. Don't wait.

If you are having hard stools, try over the counter feces conditioners or attempt one tablespoon of mineral oil, olive oil, or flaxseed oil.

Diagnosis

Endoscopy: There are numerous tools for examining belly problems. The most typical is the endoscopy. The treatment does need intravenous sedation and also takes about 30-- 45 mins; the endoscope is put through the mouth and even can envision the whole swallowing tube, belly, and duodenum. The treatment likewise enables the physician to acquire biopsy samples. In a lot of cases of blood loss, the surgeon can use the endoscope to deal with the source of hemorrhaging with laser, clips, or various other injectable drugs.

X rays: Other radiological research studies frequently made use of to assess clients with chronic belly problems include barium ingest, where a dye is taken in, and also photos of the esophagus and tummy are gotten every couple of mins. Various other examinations include 24-hour pH research, CT scans or MRI, etc.

Introduction To Gastric Sleeve

51

Sleeve gastrectomy is a medical weight-loss treatment in which the tummy is reduced to about 15% of its original size, by surgical elimination of a considerable section of the belly along the higher curvature. The outcome is a sleeve or tube-like framework. The procedure ultimately reduces the dimension of the stomach, although there could be some dilatation of the tummy in the future in life. The treatment is generally done laparoscopically as well as is irreversible.

Procedure

Sleeve gastrectomy was initially done as an alteration to another bariatric procedure, the duodenal button, and then later on, as the very first part of a two-stage stomach bypass operation on very overweight people for whom the risk of carrying out coronary stomach bypass was regarded too big. The first fat burning in these people was so effective it started to be explored as a stand-alone procedure.

Sleeve gastrectomy is the most commonly carried out bariatric surgical treatment worldwide. In several cases, sleeve gastrectomy is as efficient as gastric coronary bypass, including enhancements in sugar homeostasis before substantial weight loss has taken place. This weight-loss independent benefit is related to the reduction in stomach quantity, modifications in digestive tract peptides, and also an expression of genetics involved in sugar absorption.

The treatment includes a longitudinal resection of the belly starting from the antrum at the point 5-- 6 centimeters from the pylorus as well as finishing at the fundus near the cardia. The staying gastric sleeve is calibrated with a bougie. Many specialists choose to utilize a bougie in between 36-40 Fr with the procedure, and the suitable approximate remaining size of the stomach after the process is about 150 mL.

Stomach Sleeve Surgical procedure brings profound changes to life!

- Generally boosted lifestyle
- Excess weight reduction of concerning 60-70% within one year of surgery
- Remission or improvement of obesity-related health problems such as diabetic issues Mellitus type II, high blood pressure, rest apnea, fatty liver condition, joint discomfort, and also hyperlipidemia
- Desire to consume declines
- Reduction in hunger feeling

How Stomach Sleeve surgical treatment is carried out

1. Small cuts are made in the stomach wall surface for the insertion of tiny trocars

2. The stomach is examined, and the capillary to the lateral side of the belly is divided

3. A Bougie tube is placed into the tummy as well as serves as a sizer for the new tummy

4. The stapler is utilized to separate the belly right into two components

5. The continual firing of the stapler is made use of to divide the tummy

6. The stomach is wholly separated right into two components

7. The brand-new banana formed stomach has about 20-25% of initial stomach quantity

Exactly how does the Gastric Sleeve surgical procedure job?

1. There is a decrease in tummy volume, triggering individuals to feel full much quicker after the surgery

2. Hormone adjustments such as decreased secretion of hunger hormones trigger individuals to feel much less starving

3. Raised tummy mobility, which allows food to pass the stomach and intestinal tract quicker after surgical procedure

History and Trend of the Stomach Sleeve

At first, the Stomach Sleeve was the restrictive part of the biliopancreatic diversion duodenal switch procedure. After that, the gastric sleeve ended up being the first stage operation for very obese clients that undertook the duodenal button procedure to decrease the perioperative risks. Some people lost adequate weight after the stomach sleeve surgical procedure and also did not go through the scheduled 2nd phase duodenal button operation. These findings triggered bariatric cosmetic surgeons to consider the stomach sleeve surgery as a standalone bariatric treatment. The very first laparoscopic Stomach Sleeve was executed in 2000.

Over the past years, the variety of stomach sleeve surgical procedures continues to rise virtually yearly. Now, more than half of all bariatric surgical treatments performed in the US are gastric sleeve procedures.

Diet Plan For Gastric Bypass

The importance of diet

Gastric bypass is except every person. You need first to recognize the risks and also advantages entailed. Those that are eligible usually are more than 100 extra pounds overweight or have a body mass index (BMI) over 40. You may additionally be qualified if your BMI is between 35 and 40, and also, your health and wellness go to danger as a result of your weight. To be a practical candidate, you must likewise prepare to relearn your dietary habits. New nutritional routines can help the surgical procedure have favorable and lifelong impacts.

Before your surgical treatment, you need to make plans for a unique diet regimen to comply with before. After the surgical procedure, The presurgery diet regimen is geared in the direction of reducing the amount of fat around your liver. This decreases the threat of problems throughout the surgical procedure. After the surgical procedure, your doctor with tailor the general diet regimen standards to you. The diet regimen contains numerous weekly stages. It assists you to recoup, fulfill the needs of your now-smaller stomach, and also obtain healthier consuming routines.

Diet regimen before your surgery.

Losing weight before surgery helps reduce the amount of fat around your liver as well as the abdominal area. This might permit you to have a laparoscopy instead of open surgical treatment. Laparoscopic surgery is much less intrusive. It needs a lot less healing time and is easier on your body. Slimming down before surgical therapy not just maintains you safer during the procedure, yet it additionally assists educate you for a new way of consuming. It is a permanent modification.

Your doctor will undoubtedly establish your specific eating strategy and preop fat burning goal. Your eating plan might start as quickly as you are removed for the procedure. If sufficient fat burning does not happen, the treatment may be canceled or delayed. So, you must start the diet strategy as quickly as you can.

Instructions

Standards vary from person to person, but might include the following:

- Get rid of or reduce hydrogenated fats, consisting of entire milk items, fatty meat, as well as fried food.

- Remove or decrease foods that are high in carbohydrates, such as sweet treats, pasta, potatoes, bread, and also bread items.

- Get rid of high-sugar drinks, such as juice and also sodas.

- Exercise section control.

- Prevent binge consumption.

- Do not smoke cigarettes.

- Avoid alcohol and also leisure medications.

- Don't consume beverages with your dishes.

- Take a daily multivitamin.

- Take healthy protein supplements like protein shakes or powder.

What to eat

The pre-op diet regimen consists mostly of protein trembles as well as various other high-protein, low-calorie foods that are simple to digest. Healthy protein assists in strengthening and also shield muscle mass tissue. This can aid your body burn fat rather than muscular tissue for gas. Protein likewise aids keep your body healthy, which can accelerate recovery.

As the day for your surgery nears, you may need to follow a mostly-liquid or liquid-only diet. Based on your weight and general wellness, your physician might permit you to eat some solids throughout this moment. These could include fish, diminished hot grain, or soft-boiled eggs. Before the surgery, see to it you speak with the anesthesiologist for instructions concerning what you can or can't have before the surgical treatment These ideas are transforming. They might want you to consume carbohydrate-rich liquids up to two hours before surgery.

Diet after your surgery.

After surgical treatment, the diet plan undergoes several stages. For how long each phase lasts and also what you can be figured out by your doctor or dietitian. All stages stress the importance of section control. This practice will help you continue to drop weight and prepare you for how you will undoubtedly eat for the rest of your life.

Phase one: Fluid diet regimen

Throughout stage one, your dietary intake is geared in the direction of aiding your body to recover from surgical treatment. Your diet plan can help you stay clear of postoperative issues. For the first few days, you are only permitted to consume alcohol a few ounces of clear liquids at a time. This aids your stomach recover without being stretched out by the food. After clear fluids, you will finish to new types of fluid. These consist of:

- decaffeinated coffee and tea
- skim milk
- thin soup as well as broth
- unsweetened juice
- sugar-free jelly

- sugar-free popsicles

Stage two: Pureed diet

When your physician chooses you to prepare, you can move on to the present two. This phase contains pureed foods that have a thick, pudding-like consistency. Many foods can be mixed at home with a food processor, blender or food processor, or another gadget.

Spicy seasonings may aggravate the tummy, so stay clear of these entirely or try them individually. Prevent fruits that have great deals of seeds, such as strawberries or kiwi. You ought to also stay away from foods that are too coarse to melt, such as broccoli as well as cauliflower.

Stage three: Soft diet regimen

You will most likely consume only pureed food for several weeks. Once your medical professional decides you prepare, you can begin developing soft, easy-to-chew foods right into your diet plan. These might consist of:

- soft-boiled eggs
- ground meat
- prepared white fish
- canned fruits, such as peaches or pears

It is essential to eat little attacks. Use excellent portion control and also eat a little at a time.

Phase four: Stabilization

Stage four of the gastric bypass diet consists of the reintroduction of solid food. It usually starts concerning two months after surgical treatment. You will still need to dice or slice your food into tiny attacks because your stomach is much smaller sized. Large pieces of food may trigger a blockage. An obstruction can cause pain, nausea, or vomiting, as well as vomiting. Present foods slowly. By doing this, you can best figure out which ones your stomach can endure and which ones to avoid. Eliminate any kind of food that triggers abdominal discomfort, vomiting, or queasiness.

Foods to stay clear of in phase 4

Particular foods need not be attempted yet, such as foods that are difficult to absorb. These consist of:

- fibrous or stringy veggies, such as pea pods
- snacks
- corn on the cob
- carbonated beverages, such as seltzer
- challenging meat
- fried food
- crunchy foods, such as pretzels, granola, seeds, and also nuts

- dried out fruit

- bread and bread products, such as muffins

Concerning four months after surgical procedure, you may have the ability to resume consuming usually.

Nevertheless, section control is still crucial. Make sure your diet regimen consists primarily of fruits, veggies, lean, healthy protein, and healthy carbs. Stay clear of unhealthy foods that are high in fat, carbs, as well as calories. Consuming well means you can take pleasure in ongoing health without putting weight back on.

1. Bariatric Friendly - Tuna Patties

Time: 15 minutes

Servings: 3

Offering Dimension: 3.5 ounces

Stage: 5 Post-Op (Solid Foods).

ACTIVE INGREDIENTS:

- Tuna, canned, prepared - 225 grams or 8 oz.
- Egg, white - 2 huge (66 grams).
- Parsley, fresh leaves, cut - 1 tablespoon (2 grams)(can change with 1/4 tsp dried out parsley).
- Panko bread crumbs - 3 tablespoons (11 grams).
- Sea salt - 1/4 tsp.
- Garlic powder - 1/4 tsp.
- Olive oil - 1 tablespoon (14 grams).

INSTRUCTIONS:

1. Drain the tuna as well as include it a big dish together with the egg whites, parsley, panko bread crumbs, sea salt, and garlic powder. Mix gently with a spoon till well integrated.

2. Separate the mix into six portions and use your hands to develop little patties out of each. Make sure they behave and limited on the brink. You can place them on a reducing board when prepared.

3. Place a considerable frying pan over medium heat. Once warm, include the olive oil and also very carefully position the patties on the container. Cook for 2-3 min on each side and afterward turn off the warmth. If you're frying pan is not big enough to fit them, all you may require to do two rounds, so divide the olive oil as needed.

4. Offer and delight in!

* Note: Divide equally by the detailed variety of offers remains fresh in the freezer for three days. You may offer the patties with 1 tbsp of level, non-fat Greek yogurt if desired.

NOURISHMENT REALITIES per offering:

- Calories 130.
- Healthy protein 17 grams.
- Carbs 3 grams.
- Fat 5 grams.
- Fiber 0 grams.
- Sugar 0 grams.
- Iron 8% DV.
- Calcium 2% DV.

- Sodium 18% DV.

Nutritional expert notes: The patties obtain damp when prepared in the oil, but if you wish to add even more wetness than dip them in a bit of catsup or greek yogurt.

2. Chocolate Mousse Dip

This Delicious Chocolate Fruit Dip is a dip that people of all ages will undoubtedly love! It is just one of those dips that's so excellent you may not also care a lot about the fruit, you'll wish to get a spoon and dive in simply. I love precisely how this fruit dip dish is the best reward for any occasion or celebration, and you can make it all year. It's always a party favored, and also it will quickly disappear in no time! Plus, it just requires a few simple ingredients you may already carry hand.

This dip has such a pleasantly rich chocolatey taste, and it may be a splurge, but at the very least, you are getting lots of fresh fruit with it. So it defeats consuming a big slice of cheesecake. Plus, it tastes like cheesecake. Win-win. It will additionally provide you that chocolate-covered strawberry taste when you offer it with strawberries, and who does not enjoy chocolate-covered fruits?? Trust me; you have got to try this dip quickly!

Ingredients

Below is what you'll need for this recipe:

- Whipping cream
- Powdered sugar
- Cream cheese
- Unsweetened cocoa powder

- Vanilla extract

INSTRUCTIONS

1.   Beat the cream until soft peaks create.

2.   Add 2 tbsps powdered sugar to the cream and continue defeating till stiff optimal form.

3.   In a different mixing dish, beat lotion cheese, more powdered sugar, cacao powder, and vanilla till smooth.

4.   Mix in the cream, along with the staying powdered sugar.

Can This Chocolate Fruit Dip be Made ahead of time?

You can make this lotion cheese fruit dip as much as 4 hours ahead of time. After four hours, the fruit dip will end up being much less fluffy.

What Fruits Should I use with This Fruit Dip?

I like it most beautiful with strawberries as well as bananas. But I think raspberries would undoubtedly be another tasty option. And also, I ask yourself exactly how a citrus fruit would certainly taste with this, such as tangerines or oranges?

Tips for the Best Fruit Dip

- The cream cheese must be softened to space temperature. Otherwise, it won't whip up effectively.

- Feel free to downsize on the amount of powdered sugar you include in this recipe if you like a tangier fruit dip
- Double-check that your cocoa powder is bitter.

3. Yogurt Breakfast Popsicles

SERVINGS: 6

Planning time: 5 minutes

Freeze time: 4 hours

INGREDIENTS

- 1 cup Greek yogurt, plain, non-fat
- ½ cup milk 1% or skim
- ½ cup customary or moment oats
- 1 cup blended berries or slashed organic products

DIRECTIONS

1. Combine the milk and yogurt.
2. Partition the blend between your popsicle molds.
3. Spot a couple of berries into each form.
4. Separation of the ½ cup cereal among each shape.
5. Spot a wooden frozen yogurt stick into each shape and spot the popsicles into the cooler for at any rate 4 hours before eating.
6. To evacuate the popsicles, run the hill under a little high temp water until they come free.

NUTRITIONAL VALUES

- Serving size: 1 popsicle
- Calories: 75
- Fat: 0.6 grams
- Cholesterol: 3 milligrams
- Sodium: 36 milligrams
- Starches: 11 grams
- Dietary Fiber: 1.5 grams
- Sugar: 4 grams
- Protein: 5 grams

4. Shrimp Ceviche

SERVINGS: 4

Planning time: 25 minutes

INGREDIENTS

- 1 pound medium crude shrimp
- 1 cup lime juice (roughly five crisp limes)
- Four medium tomatoes (Roma or Italian), diced OR 8 ounces canned, diced tomatoes
- One little red onion, stripped, finely cleaved (roughly ¾ cup hacked)
- One pack cilantro stemmed and finely hacked
- Two serrano bean stew peppers, ribs and seeds expelled, minced (discretionary)

Tip: For a gentle alternative, attempt half of a medium green chime pepper.

DIRECTIONS

1. In a bowl, consolidate shrimp and lime juice.

2. Cover and marinate for around 10 to 15 minutes or until shading changes to pink. Try not to marinate excessively long, as the shrimp will "overcook" and toughen.

3. Include onions, tomatoes, bean stew peppers, and cilantro.

4. Delicately mix to consolidate.

5. Season with salt to taste.

6. Serve cold.

NUTRITIONAL VALUES

- Serving size: 4 ounces
- Calories: 160
- Fat: 1 gram
- Cholesterol: 220 milligrams
- Sodium: 265 milligrams
- Sugars: 13 grams
- Dietary Fiber: 2 grams
- Sugar: 5 grams
- Protein: 25 grams

5. Chicken Caprese

SERVINGS: 4

Planning time: 20 minutes

INGREDIENTS

- 1 pound boneless, skinless chicken bosoms
- One tablespoon olive oil
- One teaspoon dry Italian flavoring (or equivalent pieces of garlic powder, dried oregano, and dried basil)
- Four thick (½-inch) cuts a ready tomato
- Four 1-ounce cuts new mozzarella cheddar
- Three tablespoons balsamic vinegar
- Two tablespoons daintily cut basil
- Pepper to taste

DIRECTIONS

1. Warmth a flame broil or barbecue dish over medium-high warmth.

2. Shower 1 tablespoon of olive oil over chicken bosoms and season to taste with and pepper.

3. Sprinkle Italian flavoring over the chicken.

4. Spot the chicken on the flame broil and cook for 3 to 5 minutes for each side, or until done. Cook time

will differ contingent upon the thickness of your chicken bosoms.

5. At the point when chicken is done, top with a cut of mozzarella cheddar and cook for one increasingly minute.

6. Expel from warmth and spot chicken bosoms on a plate.

7. Top each bosom with one cut of tomato, meagerly cut basil, and pepper to taste.

8. Sprinkle with balsamic vinegar or balsamic coating and serve.

NUTRITIONAL VALUES

- Serving size: 6 ounces (4 ounces chicken with 1 ounce tomato and 1 ounce cheddar)
- Calories: 230
- Fat: 9 gram
- Cholesterol: 80 milligrams
- Sodium: 105 milligrams
- Sugars: 4 grams
- Dietary Fiber: 0 grams
- Sugar: 2.5 grams
- Protein: 33 grams

6. Dark Bean and Corn Salad

SERVINGS: 6

INGREDIENTS

- 1 cup corn, the entire part
- Two jars (16 ounces each) dark beans, flushed and depleted
- ¼ cup parsley slashed new
- Two tablespoons red onion, minced
- ¼ cup balsamic vinegar
- Two tablespoon olive oil
- One teaspoon lemon juice
- One teaspoon garlic, minced
- One teaspoon nectar or dark-colored sugar
- Run salt
- ¼ teaspoon ground dark pepper

DIRECTIONS

1. Blend crisp corn, dark beans, red onion, and fresh parsley in a large blending bowl.
2. Whisk together balsamic vinegar, olive oil, lemon juice, garlic, nectar, salt, and pepper.
3. Pour over dark beans and corn blend.

4. Let the plate of mixed greens marinade for 30 minutes before serving.

NUTRITIONAL VALUES

- Serving size: ½ cup
- Calories: 160
- Fat: 5 grams
- Cholesterol: 0 milligrams
- Potassium: 306 milligrams
- Sodium: 40 milligrams
- Starches: 23 grams
- Dietary Fiber: 6 grams
- Sugars: 3 grams
- Protein: 6 grams

7. Nut Applesauce Chicken

SERVINGS: 8

Planning time: 10 minutes

Cook time: 60 minutes

INGREDIENTS

- 2½ pounds chicken pieces
- ¼ cup yellow mustard
- ⅛ cup Splenda dark colored sugar unloaded
- ½ cup powdered peanuts
- Salt and pepper to taste
- 1 (15 ounces) container fruit purée, unsweetened

DIRECTIONS

1. Cook chicken in sauté container.
2. When approaching thoroughly cooked, include fruit purée, mustard, dark colored sugar, and powdered peanuts.
3. Mix ingredients together.
4. Stew over medium warmth until an inward temperature of 165ºF is come to.

NUTRITIONAL VALUES

- Serving size: 2 tablespoons
- Calories: 50

- Fat: 2 grams
- Cholesterol: 60 milligrams
- Sodium: 203 milligrams
- Sugars: 13 grams
- Dietary Fiber: 2 grams
- Sugar: 10 grams
- Protein: 3 grams

8. Hot Peanut Vegetarian Chili

SERVINGS: 10 – 12

You won't miss the meat right now, stew, made with powdered peanuts.

INGREDIENTS

- One tablespoon nut oil (or canola oil)
- 1 cup hacked onion
- Two cloves garlic, minced
- Two tablespoons stew powder
- One teaspoon chipotle stew pepper (discretionary)
- ¼ teaspoon dried oregano
- One can (16 ounces) dark beans, depleted and washed
- One can (16 ounces) white beans, drained and washed
- ⅔ cup powdered peanuts
- One can (28 ounces) diced tomato
- One can (15 ounces) tomato sauce
- 2 cups vegetable soup

DIRECTIONS

1. In a solid Dutch stove, heat oil over medium-high warmth.

2. Include onion and garlic, sauté 3 – 4 minutes, or until delicate.

3. Mix in stew powder, pepper, oregano, and salt.

4. Sauté 2 minutes or until fragrant.

5. Include beans, corn, powdered peanuts, tomatoes, tomato sauce, and soup.

6. Heat to the point of boiling.

7. Decrease heat and stew for 30 minutes.

Note: This formula might be cooked in the moderate cooker for 2 – 3 hours.

NUTRITIONAL VALUES

- Serving size: ½ cup
- Calories: 125
- Fat: 2.5 grams
- Sodium: 582 milligrams
- Sugars: 22 grams
- Dietary Fiber: 7 grams
- Sugar: 5 grams
- Protein: 8 grams

9. Nutty spread and Jelly Pancakes

SERVINGS: 4

INGREDIENTS

- ½ cup low-fat curds
- ½ cup moment cereal
- Two tablespoons powdered peanuts
- Four enormous egg whites
- 1 cup solidified blended berry mix

DIRECTIONS

1. Put Items in a blender in a specific order: curds, corn, powdered peanuts, and egg whites.

2. Turn on blender and mix until smooth like hotcake player.

3. Fill a bowl and overlap in berry organic product blend.

4. Use cooking shower in skillet. Makes 4 to 7 hotcakes relying upon size.

NUTRITIONAL VALUES

- Serving size: 1 flapjack
- Calories: 90
- Fat: 1.5 grams
- Cholesterol: 1 milligrams

- Sodium: 195 milligrams
- Starches: 9 grams
- Dietary Fiber: 1.5 grams
- Sugar: 1 grams
- Protein: 10 grams

10. Nut Powder Salad Dressing

SERVINGS: 2

This lower-calorie, Asian-motivated nut dressing made with powdered nutty spread is fabulous as a plunging sauce or plate of mixed greens dressing.

INGREDIENTS

- Two tablespoons powdered peanuts
- One tablespoon soy sauce, low sodium
- One tablespoon water
- ⅛ teaspoon garlic powder
- ¼ teaspoon ground pepper
- ¼ teaspoon Szechuan bean stew sauce
- One teaspoon Splenda darker sugar mix
- ⅛ teaspoon sesame oil

DIRECTIONS

1. Mix all ingredients well and serve. Refrigerate any remaining sauce.

NUTRITIONAL VALUES

- Serving size: 2 tablespoons
- Calories: 50
- Starches: 7 grams
- Sodium: 562 milligrams

- Fat: 2 grams
- Protein: 3 grams
- Dietary Fiber: 1 grams
- Sugar: 5 grams

11. Pumpkin-Ricotta Protein Pie

SERVINGS: 12

INGREDIENTS

- 2 cups 100% unadulterated pumpkin puree, canned, without salt

- Two eggs, huge

- 1 cup milk, nonfat (skim milk)

- 1 cup ricotta cheddar, part-skim

- ⅓ cup Truvia for Baking or Splenda Sugar Blend

- Two scoops 100% Unflavored Whey Protein Isolate, (for example, BiPro 1 scoop=~22 grams)

- ½ teaspoon salt

- One teaspoon cinnamon, ground

- One teaspoon nutmeg, ground

- 2-ounce bundle walnut parts

DIRECTIONS

1. Preheat stove to 350ºF.

2. Splash 9-inch pie dish and four little ramekins with nonstick shower.

3. Mix ricotta cheddar, eggs, and ½ cup of milk until smooth; it ought to be fluid-like.

4. Include remaining ingredients and mix until smooth.

5. Empty fluid blend into the splashed cooking dish, design with walnuts on top.

6. Prepare for 40 – 45 minutes or until the center is set and genuinely healthy. It ought not to shake when thoroughly cooked. The sides and focus should dark-colored and grow up to twofold its size. On the off chance that you experience over-sautéing on the top, diminish temperature to 325ºF for the rest of the time.

7. Chill for 1 hour before cutting. This likewise considers the pie extension to settle.

8. Cut into 12 even pieces with a stainless blade. Wipe the knife between each cut for a well put together.

Tip: If you choose to utilize outside, (for example, graham saltine, or a customary pie baked good, you should alter the nourishment data and calories upwards in like manner.

NUTRITIONAL VALUES

- Serving Size: One cut of pie after it's cut into 12 pieces
- Calories: 105
- Cholesterol: 33 milligrams
- Sugars: 10 grams
- Sodium: 151 milligrams
- Fat: 3.5 grams

- Protein: 6 grams
- Dietary Fiber: 2 grams
- Sugar: 8 grams

12. High-Protein Pumpkin Pie Oatmeal

SERVINGS: 1

INGREDIENTS

- ⅓ cup old-fashioned oats (30 grams)
- ½ cup pumpkin, canned
- ⅛ teaspoon cinnamon
- Run ground cloves
- Run ground ginger
- One teaspoon Truvia preparing mix
- ½ cup no salt included 1% curds

DIRECTIONS

1. Consolidate oats, pumpkin, flavors, and sugar in a microwave-safe bowl.
2. Microwave on high for 90 seconds.
3. Mix in the curds.
4. Microwave on high for 60 seconds.
5. Let sit for two or three minutes before eating.

NUTRITIONAL VALUES

- Calories: 205
- Cholesterol: 3 milligrams
- Starches: 34 grams
- Sodium: 312 milligrams

- Fat: 3 grams
- Protein: 14 grams
- Dietary Fiber: 7 grams
- Sugar: 9 grams

13. Apple and Tuna Sandwiches Recipe

SERVINGS: 3

INGREDIENTS

- One can fish, pressed in water (6.5 ounces, depleted)
- One apple
- ¼ cup yogurt, low-fat vanilla
- One teaspoon mustard
- ½ teaspoon nectar
- Six cuts entire wheat bread
- Three lettuces leave

DIRECTIONS

1. Wash and strip the apple. Cleave it into little pieces.
2. Channel the water from the container of fish.
3. Put the fish, apple, yogurt, mustard, and nectar in a medium bowl. Mix well.
4. Spread ½ cup of the fish blend onto every three cuts of bread.
5. Top the sandwich with a lettuce leaf and a cut of bread.

NUTRITIONAL VALUES

- Serving size: ? of formula
- Calories: 250
- Cholesterol: 28 miligrams
- Starches: 30 grams
- Sodium: 330 milligrams
- Fat: 2.5 grams
- Protein: 23 grams
- Dietary Fiber: 5 grams
- Sugar: 5.25 grams

14. Prepared Chicken With Vegetables

SERVINGS: 6

INGREDIENTS

- Four potatoes, cut
- Six carrots, cut
- One huge onion, quartered
- One chicken, crude, cut into pieces with skin expelled
- ½ cup of water
- One teaspoon thyme
- ¼ teaspoon pepper

DIRECTIONS

1. Preheat stove to 400 degrees.
2. Spot potatoes, carrots, and onions in a large broiling container.
3. Put chicken pieces on the vegetables.
4. Blend water, thyme, and pepper. Pour over chicken and vegetables.
5. Spoon squeezes over chicken on more than one occasion during cooking.
6. Heat for one hour or more until cooked and delicate.

NUTRITIONAL VALUES

- Serving size: ? of formula
- Calories: 240
- Sugar: 25 grams
- Sugar: 10 grams
- Fat: 3.5 grams
- Protein: 26 grams
- Sodium: 130 milligrams
- Fiber: 4 grams

15. Luxurious Chocolate Soy Dessert Recipe

SERVINGS: 8

Planning Time: 10 minutes

Chill Time: 30 minutes

Complete Time: 40 minutes

INGREDIENTS

- One envelope unflavored gelatin
- ¼ cup of heated water
- One bundle (1.4 oz) without sugar, sans fat chocolate fudge moment pudding
- 1 cup cold skim milk
- 16 ounces smooth tofu
- ½ teaspoon vanilla concentrate
- One tablespoon cocoa powder (discretionary)
- ¼ teaspoon peppermint extricate (discretionary)

DIRECTIONS

1. In a little bowl, blend the heated water and unflavored gelatin. Put in a safe spot and permit to the firm.
2. In a medium-sized bowl, consolidate the virus skim milk and moment pudding blend.

3. Bones the tofu into ½-to 1-inch 3D shapes and spot in a bowl with pudding blend. Rapidly whisk together to separate the soy shapes.

4. Include the vanilla concentrate and discretionary cocoa powder and peppermint remove.

5. Spoon the pudding and tofu blend into a blender or nourishment processor. Mix until smooth. You may need to mix for around 5 seconds and hand blend or shake the substance with the goal that the engine doesn't stick.

6. When the blend has a smoothie-like surface, progressively include the gelatin until very much joined and mix once more.

7. Fill a glass 8-inch dish, spread and spot in the fridge for in any event 30 minutes to firm. The more it sits, the firmer it will turn into.

8. Cut into eight segments and appreciate it!

NUTRITIONAL VALUES

- Serving size: ½ cup or 2-inch square
- Calories: 56
- Sugar: 6 grams
- Fat: 1 grams (0 grams immersed)
- Protein: 5 grams
- Cholesterol: 1 milligram

- Sodium: 181 milligrams
- Fiber: 0 grams

16. Pork and Black Bean Verde Stew Recipe

SERVINGS: 4

INGREDIENTS

- Two teaspoons extra-virgin olive oil
- 1 pound pork flank or tenderloin, cut back of unmistakable excess and cut into 1" 3D squares
- 1¼ cup cleaved onions
- Three cloves garlic
- Two canned chipotle peppers in sauce, minced in addition to 1 teaspoon adobo sauce
- One teaspoon ground cumin
- One parcel Goya Sazon with coriander and annatto (or comparative flavoring bundle)
- One can (14 ounces) no salt included chicken stock
- One can (14.5 ounces) no salt added diced tomatoes in juice
- One can (14.5 ounces) no salt included dark beans, depleted and flushed
- One teaspoon squashed red pepper pieces (discretionary)

DIRECTIONS

1. An enormous pot or Dutch broiler, heat olive oil over medium-high warmth.

2. Include pork solid shapes and cook, blending every so often for 4-6 minutes or until caramelized on all sides.

3. Include onion and garlic and cook for 2-3 minutes, or until beginning to mellow.

4. Include chipotle peppers and sauce, cumin, and flavoring parcel. Mix to blend.

5. Include stock, tomatoes, beans, and red pepper drop whenever wanted. Mix to blend well.

6. Heat stew to the point of boiling at that point diminishes warmth to low.

7. Spread pot and stew for 45 minutes to 60 minutes, or until the port is fork delicate.

8. Serve stew in astounds dark colored rice or add rice to stew, whenever wanted. (Rice excluded from nutritional examination.)

NUTRITIONAL VALUES

- Serving size: ¼ of formula, excluding rice
- Calories: 308
- Sugar: 25 grams
- Fat: 7 grams (2 grams immersed)
- Protein: 33 grams
- Cholesterol: 84 milligrams
- Sodium: 414 milligrams

- Fiber: 6 grams

17. Asian Chicken Lettuce Wraps Recipe

SERVINGS: 4

INGREDIENTS

- One can (8 ounces) bamboo shoots, depleted and minced
- One can (8 ounces) water chestnuts, consumed and minced
- Three tablespoons sherry cooking wine
- Two tablespoons hoisin sauce
- One tablespoon unsalted nutty spread
- Two teaspoons low-sodium soy sauce
- Two teaspoons hot pepper sauce, for example, Sriracha
- Two parcels (.035 ounce each) sugar substitute, (for example, Splenda)
- One tablespoon minced garlic
- 1 cup minced onion
- ½ pound ground chicken bosom
- One teaspoon minced ginger
- ¼ teaspoon salt
- One teaspoon toasted sesame oil
- Eight little leaves margarine lettuce

- One entire green onion, cleaved
- 1 small cucumber, cut into 1" strips

DIRECTIONS

1. In a medium bowl, join the bamboo shoots, water chestnuts, sherry, hoisin sauce, nutty spread, soy sauce, hot-pepper sauce, and sugar substitute. Blend well. Put in a safe spot.

2. Fog a large, nonstick skillet with cooking splash and set over medium warmth.

3. Include the onion and cook for 4 minutes or until onions are fragrant and mellowed.

4. Include the garlic and cook for brief more.

5. Increment the warmth to medium-high and include the ground chicken, ginger, and salt.

6. Cook, separating the chicken with a spatula or wooden spoon, for 3 to 4 minutes, until never again pink.

7. Include the bamboo shoot and water chestnut blend.

8. Cook for 2 minutes, or until warmed through.

9. Mix in the toasted sesame oil.

10. Expel the skillet from the warmth.

11. To serve, isolate the chicken blend evening onto every one of the eight lettuce leaves.

12. Top with cleaved green onion and cucumber. Serve right away.

NUTRITIONAL VALUES

- Serving size: 2 lettuce wraps
- Calories: 155
- Cholesterol: 33 milligrams
- Starches: 11 grams
- Sodium: 637 milligrams
- Fat: 4 grams
- Protein: 16 grams
- Dietary Fiber: 5 grams
- Sugar: 4 grams

18. Asian Chicken Lettuce Wraps Recipe

SERVINGS: 4

INGREDIENTS

- One can (8 ounces) bamboo shoots, depleted and minced
- One can (8 ounces) water chestnuts, depleted and minced
- Three tablespoons sherry cooking wine
- Two tablespoons hoisin sauce
- One tablespoon unsalted nutty spread
- Two teaspoons low-sodium soy sauce
- Two teaspoons hot pepper sauce, for example, Sriracha
- Two bundles (.035 ounce each) sugar substitute, (for example, Splenda)
- One tablespoon minced garlic
- 1 cup minced onion
- ½ pound ground chicken bosom
- One teaspoon minced ginger
- ¼ teaspoon salt
- One teaspoon toasted sesame oil
- Eight little leaves spread lettuce

- One entire green onion, cleaved
- 1 small cucumber cut into 1" strips

DIRECTIONS

1. In a medium bowl, consolidate the bamboo shoots, water chestnuts, sherry, hoisin sauce, nutty spread, soy sauce, hot-pepper sauce, and sugar substitute. Blend well. Put in a safe spot.

2. Fog a huge, nonstick skillet with cooking splash and set over medium warmth.

3. Include the onion and cook for 4 minutes or until onions are fragrant and relaxed.

4. Include the garlic and cook for brief more.

5. Increment the warmth to medium-high and include the ground chicken, ginger, and salt.

6. Cook, separating the chicken with a spatula or wooden spoon, for 3 to 4 minutes, until never again pink.

7. Include the bamboo shoot and water chestnut blend.

8. Cook for 2 minutes, or until warmed through.

9. Mix in the toasted sesame oil.

10. Expel the skillet from the warmth.

11. To serve, isolate the chicken blend evening onto every one of the eight lettuce leaves.

12. Top with hacked green onion and cucumber. Serve right away.

NUTRITIONAL VALUES

- Serving size: 2 lettuce wraps
- Calories: 155
- Cholesterol: 33 milligrams
- Starches: 11 grams
- Sodium: 637 milligrams
- Fat: 4 grams
- Protein: 16 grams
- Dietary Fiber: 5 grams
- Sugar: 4 grams

19. Chicken Cheesesteak Wrap Recipe

SERVINGS: 1

INGREDIENTS

- ¼ pound boneless, skinless chicken bosom, cut back of apparent excess
- ¼ cup onions, hacked
- ¼ cup green pepper, cut
- ¼ cup mushrooms, cut
- One wedge (¾ ounce) Laughing Cow Original light swiss cheddar or equal
- One entire wheat flour, low-carb tortilla
- Two teaspoons cut cured hot stew peppers (discretionary)

DIRECTIONS

1. Spot chicken bosom on cutting board, pound to 1/4" meager and cut into exceptionally slight strips.

2. Spot a skillet over medium-high warmth and fog with cooking shower.

3. Add the onion and chicken to the warmed skillet and cook until onions are translucent and chicken is never again pink all through.

4. Add green peppers and mushrooms to the skillet and cook until peppers and mushrooms mellow.

5. Spot tortilla between 2 damp paper towels. Microwave for 20 seconds.

6. Lay the warm tortilla level and spread cheddar in an even strip in the center.

7. Top with chicken, peppers, onions, and mushrooms.

8. Include bean stew peppers if utilizing.

9. Overlap sides of tortilla over the center. Serve right away.

NUTRITIONAL VALUES

- Serving size: 1 wrap
- Calories: 264
- Sugar: 17 grams
- Fat: 6 grams (2 grams immersed)
- Protein: 33 grams
- Cholesterol: 76 milligrams
- Sodium: 620 milligrams
- Fiber: 4 grams

20. Not so much Fried Rice Recipe

SERVINGS: 2

INGREDIENTS

- Two tablespoons low-sodium soy sauce
- One teaspoon mustard
- One teaspoon stew glue
- One teaspoon toasted sesame oil
- 3 ounces boneless, skinless chicken bosom cut into ½" shapes
- Dark pepper, to taste
- ½ cup finely slashed entire green onions
- ¼ cup slashed carrot
- One clove garlic, minced
- ¾ cup cooked short-grain more colored rice
- ¼ cup solidified peas
- Two enormous egg whites
- Olive oil shower

DIRECTIONS

1. In a little bowl, join soy sauce, mustard, bean stew glue, and sesame oil. Put in a safe spot.
2. Season the cubed chicken with dark pepper.

3. Fog an enormous, nonstick wok or skillet with cooking shower and spot over medium-high warmth until it is hot enough for a drop of water to sizzle on it.

4. Dissipate the chicken solid shapes into the wok or skillet.

5. Cook, blending at times until caramelized on all sides and never again pink inside.

6. Move chicken to a plate and spread to keep warm.

7. Gently fog the wok or skillet with a cooking shower once more. Set over medium-high warmth.

8. Include the green onions, carrot, and garlic to the container.

9. Cook, blending now and again, for 2-3 minutes.

10. Include the cooked rice and peas.

11. Keep cooking and blending for 2 minutes or until the blend is hot all through.

12. Utilizing a spoon or spatula, make an opening in the rice and veggies from uncovering the focal point of the skillet.

13. Off the warmth, gently fog the uncovered piece of the skillet with cooking splash.

14. Include the egg whites and mix to blend them into the rice.

15. Cook for 1-2 minutes, or until the egg is cooked.

16. Return the chicken to the container and mix in the held soy sauce blend.

17. Leave on heat, mixing continually, for around one moment or until warmed. Serve right away.

NUTRITIONAL VALUES

- Serving size: ½ formula
- Calories: 208
- Starch: 25 grams
- Fat: 3.5 grams (1 grams soaked)
- Protein: 17 grams
- Cholesterol: 25 milligrams
- Sodium: 260 milligrams
- Fiber: 3.5 grams

21. Egg-Chilada Recipe

SERVINGS: 1

INGREDIENTS

- One egg + 1 egg white
- Dark pepper and salt to taste
- The 1-ounce protein of decision (tofu, chicken, or ground meat function admirably)
- Two tablespoons salsa, (for example, Tostito's medium)
- One tablespoon destroyed Mexican mix cheddar
- Two tablespoons plain without fat Greek yogurt

DIRECTIONS

1. Scramble the egg and egg white in a little bowl
2. Splash a skillet or frying pan with cooking shower and set it over medium warmth.
3. Pour the fried eggs onto the warmed dish and permit it to spread into a by and large round shape.
4. Disregard the eggs for a moment or two, permitting the edges to set. Include a sprinkle of dark pepper and salt to the eggs while they're setting.
5. Slide a spatula underneath the eggs and flip (don't stress if some egg pours off now).

6. Cook eggs on the opposite side around two minutes or until totally cooked and move to a plate.

7. Make a portion of filling for your egg-enchilada with 1 oz—protein of decision and Mexican cheddar.

8. Move up the egg "hotcake" to frame your egg-enchilada.

9. Top with salsa and Greek yogurt.

NUTRITIONAL VALUES

- Serving size: 1 egg-chilada
- Calories: 171
- Sugar: 3 grams
- Fat: 8 grams
- Protein: 23 grams
- Sodium: 432 milligrams
- Sugar: 3 grams

22. Cheesecake Pudding Recipe

INGREDIENTS

- 1 cup plain sans fat Greek yogurt
- One bundle sans sugar cheesecake pudding blend

DIRECTIONS

1. Join components in a blender and puree until smooth.

NUTRITIONAL VALUES

Serving size: ¼ cup

Protein: 7 grams

23. Seared Rainbow Trout Recipe

SERVINGS: 2

INGREDIENTS

- 8 ounces rainbow trout filets
- 3 Tbsp yellow cornmeal
- 1⅓ Tbsp cleaved parsley
- ¼ tsp ground celery seeds
- ¼ tsp ground dark pepper
- One squeeze salt
- 2 tsp olive oil

DIRECTIONS

1. Clean and flush fish filets. Check to ensure all bones are expelled. Pat dry.

2. Combine cornmeal, salt, pepper, celery seed, and hacked parsley.

3. Spread fish with cornmeal blend and press onto fish.

4. Warmth olive oil in a non-stick skillet. Cook fish 2 to 3 minutes for each side. Fish ought to be dark-colored and fresh and should piece when punctured with a fork.

NUTRITIONAL ANALYSIS PER SERVING (4 ounce serving)

- Serving Size: About 1 cup

- Calories: 240
- All out Fat: 10g
- All out Protein: 25g
- All out Carbohydrates: 10g
- Cholesterol: 67mg
- Sodium: 338mg
- Sugars: 0g

24. Pumpkin and Black Bean Soup Recipe

SERVINGS: 6 (around 1 cup each)

35 minutes

INGREDIENTS

- Two tablespoons olive oil
- One medium onion slashed
- Four garlic cloves, minced
- One tablespoon ground cumin
- One teaspoon bean stew powder
- ½ teaspoon dark pepper
- Two jars (15 ounces) dark beans, flushed and depleted
- 1 cup canned diced tomatoes
- 2 cups hamburger juices
- One can (16 ounces) pumpkin puree

DIRECTIONS

1. Warmth oil in a soup pot over medium warmth, sauté onions, garlic, cumin, bean stew powder, and pepper until delicate.

2. Mix in dark beans, tomatoes, juices, and pumpkin.

3. Stew revealed mixing once in a while for around 25 minutes until soup is a thick consistency

4. Fill in as may be, or puree, utilizing an inundation blender for a smooth texture.

5. Recommendations

6. Mix in plain Greek yogurt for included protein and smoothness.

7. Include ½-pound ground meat for an extra protein.

NUTRITIONAL ANALYSIS PER SERVING

- Serving Size: About 1 cup
- Calories: 290
- Complete Fat: 6g
- Complete Protein: 15g
- Absolute Carbohydrates: 46g
- Dietary Fiber: 11g
- Sugars: 3g

25. Greek Yogurt Chicken Recipe

SERVINGS: 4

INGREDIENTS

- Four boneless skinless chicken bosoms (4 oz each)
- 1 cup plain Greek yogurt
- ½ cup ground Parmesan cheddar
- One teaspoon garlic powder
- 1½ teaspoons flavoring salt
- ½ teaspoon pepper

DIRECTIONS

1. Preheat stove to 375 degrees.
2. Consolidate Greek yogurt, cheddar, and seasonings in a bowl.
3. Line preparing sheet with foil and shower with cooking splash.
4. Coat every chicken bosom in Greek yogurt blend and spot on thwarted preparing sheet.
5. Prepare for 45 minutes.
6. Appreciate!!

NUTRITIONAL ANALYSIS PER SERVING

- Absolute Calories: 266

- Absolute fat: 4g
- Soaked Fat: 3g
- Absolute sugars: 3g
- Dietary Fiber: 0g
- Sugars: 2g
- Protein: 46g

26. High-Protein Cottage Cheese Pancakes Recipe

SERVINGS: 4 hotcakes

INGREDIENTS

- ⅓ cup universally handy flour
- ½ tsp heating pop
- 1 cup low-fat curds
- ½ tablespoons canola oil
- Three eggs, softly beaten

DIRECTIONS

1. Join powder and heating soft drinks in a little bowl.
2. Join the remaining ingredients in an enormous bowl.
3. Empty flour blend into curds blend and mix until simply joined.
4. Warmth a large skillet over medium heat, cover with cooking shower.
5. Pour? Cup bits of player onto the skillet and cook until bubbles show up superficially.
6. Flip and cook until darker.
7. Present with low-calorie syrup. (Attempt Walden Farms.)

NUTRITIONAL ANALYSIS PER SERVING

- Serving Size: 1 hotcake
- Calories: 152
- Sugar: 10 g
- Fat: 7 g
- Protein: 13 g
- Sodium: 385 mg
- Sugar: 2 g

27. Thai Tofu Quinoa Bowl Recipe

SERVINGS: 6

INGREDIENTS

- One bundle additional firm tofu (15 oz), diced
- Two tablespoons soy sauce
- One tablespoon sesame oil
- 1 cup uncooked quinoa
- 1½ cups of chicken juices
- ½ cup fragmented almonds
- 1 cup destroyed carrots
- 2/3 cup slashed scallions
- ½ cup crisp cilantro
- For the sauce:
- Two teaspoons creamy, nutty spread
- Two tablespoons Sriracha sauce
- Two tablespoons rice wine vinegar
- Three tablespoons coconut milk
- ½ tablespoon dark colored sugar
- One garlic clove, minced
- ½ lime, squeezed
- One teaspoon ground ginger

INSTRUCTIONS

1. Thirty minutes before cooking, channel, and flush tofu.

2. Envelop by clean kitchen towel and spot on a rimmed supper plate.

3. Spot another plate on top and weight down with something substantial to press out a portion of the abundance fluid.

4. Let sit 15-30 minutes.

5. Preheat grill to 350? F.

6. Hurl tofu, soy sauce, and sesame oil in a bowl.

7. Spot tofu in a single layer on a lined heating sheet.

8. Heat for 35-40 minutes hurling like clockwork to fresh tofu on all sides.

9. Toast and cook quinoa.

10. Spot a medium sizes sauce skillet on medium-low warmth.

11. Include dry quinoa and toast for 5 minutes, sometimes blending until brilliant darker.

12. Add stock to quinoa, lower heat somewhat.

13. Spread and cook for 12-15 minutes or until all fluid is assimilated.

14. Cushion with a fork and put in a safe spot.

15. Make the sauce:

16. Spot nutty spread in bowl and microwave for 10 seconds to liquefy.

17. Include remaining ingredients and whisk well to consolidate.

18. Toast the almonds:

19. Spot almonds in a little sauce dish.

20. Cook on medium-low warmth, mixing at times until almonds are brilliantly developed.

21. Hurl together quinoa, vegetables, herbs, tofu, and nuts.

22. Pour sauce over everything and hurl to consolidate. Appreciate!

Nourishment FACTS (1 serving, 1/6 of formula)

- Calories: 232
- Complete Fat: 10 g
- Complete Carbohydrates: 27 g
- Dietary Fiber: 4.5 g
- Sugars: 4 g
- Protein: 12g

28. Ginger Beef Stir Fry Recipe

SERVINGS: 6

INGREDIENTS

- 1 pound flank steak
- Two teaspoons ground ginger
- Two medium garlic cloves
- 6 ounces hamburger soup (fat-free)
- ¼ cup (2 ounces) hoisin sauce
- Three tablespoons soy sauce
- One tablespoons cornstarch
- One teaspoon canola oil
- ¼ teaspoon squashed red pepper pieces
- 3 ounces broccoli florets
- ½ medium yellow, red or green ringer pepper cut into strips
- ½ cup moment dark colored rice
- Two medium stalks bok choy cut into ½-inch cuts
- 8-ounce can chop water chestnuts

Guidelines

1. In blending bowl, mix steak, garlic, and ginger. Put in a safe spot.
2. Get ready rice as per directions on the bundle.

3. Join the soup, hoisin sauce, soy sauce, and cornstarch in a bowl. Mix until broke down.

4. In wok, heat oil, and red pepper pieces over medium-high warmth.

5. Cook steak 4-5 minutes or until sautéed. Mix continually. Put in a safe spot.

6. Put broccoli, ringer pepper, and carrot into a dish. Cook over medium-high warmth for 2-3 minutes or until delicate fresh. Mix. (On the off chance that blend turns out to be excessively dry, include 1-2 tablespoons water.)

7. Mix in bok choy and water chestnuts. Cook for extra 1-2 minutes or under bok choy is delicate fresh. Mix continually.

8. Make a well in the focus of container, and pour in juices.

9. Cook 1-2 minutes or until juices thicken, every so often mixes soup.

10. Blend in hamburger. Cook 1-2 minutes or until warm.

11. Serve over rice.

Sustenance FACTS (? formula)

- Calories: 275
- Fat: 8 grams

- Sugars: 25 grams
- Dietary Fiber: 2 grams
- Sugars: 6 grams
- Protein: 17 grams

Part 2

Introduction

You are making all of the right moves to improve your lifestyle. You will surely want to add Gastric Sleeve Cookbook: Delicious Recipes to Recover Yourself After Bariatric Weight Loss Surgery to your personal library. It will provide you with many new dishes you never thought would be possible to prepare and remain healthy.

You will soon discover within the pages of this cookbook that you are truly entering a new stage of your life. You have the tools to continue down the right path to a much healthier future.

These are just a few of the recipes you can enjoy:

- Chicken Creole
- Ranch Cheddar Turkey Burgers
- Mediterranean Salmon with Pasta
- Crunchy Tuna Patties
- Curried Carrot Soup
- Meatloaf Muffins
- Caramel Apple Salad
- Coconut Meringue Cookies

Plus, so much more!

The following chapters will discuss many ways to cook food you have always eaten. You will discover how many different ways you can cook beef, poultry, seafood, and many other foods. For most of the recipes it is important to use non-fat, reduced-sodium, and similar choices when they are available, since that is how you can easily reduce the calorie and carbohydrate intakes.

There are plenty of books on this subject on the market, thanks again for choosing this one! Every effort was made to ensure it is full of as much useful information as possible. Please enjoy!

Happy Cooking!

Chapter 1: Poultry And Turkey

Almond Chicken Salad with Asparagus

Ingredients

12 ounces cooked chicken breast- boneless and skinless

2 cups asparagus tips

1 teaspoon each:

- Fresh lemon juice
- Curry powder

½ cup plain, yogurt

1/8 teaspoon pepper

¼ teaspoon salt

¼ cup freshly chopped cilantro

½ cup red bell pepper (seeded and chopped)

Spinach leaves

2 tablespoons toasted sliced almonds

Instructions

1. Diagonally cut the asparagus and chop the chicken.
2. Steam the asparagus for two minutes.

3. Mix the lemon juice, salt, curry, pepper, and yogurt. Blend in the chicken asparagus, almonds, and cilantro. Toss to cover evenly and serve over the leaves of spinach.

Yields: Four servings

Cal: 161.5 | P: 24 g | C: 7.9 g | F: 4.1 g

Baked Chicken and Vegetables

Ingredients

6 sliced carrots

4 sliced potatoes

1 large quartered onion

1 skinless raw chicken

1 teaspoon thyme

½ cup water

¼ teaspoon pepper

Instructions

1. Set the oven temperature in advance to 400ºF.
2. Arrange the carrots, potatoes, and onions in a roasting pan. Add the chicken last.
3. Combine the pepper, thyme, and water. Dump them over the ingredients in the pan.
4. Bake for one hour until brown and tender. Baste the chicken with the juices several times.

Yields: Six servings

Cal: 240 | P: 26 g | C: 25 g | F: 3.5g

Brown Sugar Garlic Chicken

Ingredients

12 ounces chicken breasts (no skins or bones)

1 garlic clove

2 tablespoons butter

Dash of black pepper

4 teaspoons brown sugar

Instructions

1. Melt the butter and add the garlic in a frying pan.
2. Add the chicken flavored with the pepper, and cook until done (about 15 minutes).
3. Sprinkle with the brown sugar, cook for five minutes, and serve.

Yields: Four servings

Cal: 166.4 | P: 19.4 g | C: 4.3 g | F: 8.0 g

Chicken and Broccoli Casserole

Ingredients

1 package broccoli spears (frozen - 10 ounces)

1 pound breast of chicken

1 can of (low sodium) cream of mushroom soup

3 tbsp. mayonnaise

1 cup shredded cheddar cheese

Instructions

1. Remove all bones and skin from the chicken. Boil and drain the chicken breasts. When cooled, cut into one-inch bits.
2. Add the soup and mayonnaise in a casserole dish. Blend in the chicken and broccoli, mixing well.
3. Dust with the cheese and bake for approximately twenty minutes.

Yields: Four servings

Cal: 284.2 | P: 36.8 g | C: 15.8 g | F: 7.3 g

Chicken Broccoli and Tomato Stir Fry

Ingredients

1 pound chicken breast (boneless - chopped

1 tbsp. soy sauce

2 tsp. canola oil

1 tsp. fresh ginger

¼ tsp. salt

2 tsp. finely chopped garlic

3 cups broccoli florets

4 firm plum tomatoes

1 cup (divided) reduced-sodium chicken broth

1 tbsp. cornstarch

Instructions

1. Cut the chicken into one-inch chunks.
2. Finely chop the garlic and ginger. You can substitute fresh ginger with ¼ teaspoon ground ginger. Slice lengthwise and quarter the tomatoes.
3. Use a pan over med-high heat or use a wok to warm the oil. Place the chopped breast of chicken into the pan/wok and cook three minutes.
4. Empty the soy sauce, ginger, and garlic into the pan while stirring; add the broccoli and one-half cup of

the broth. Place a lid on the pan and continue cooking for two to three more minutes.
5. Mix the remainder of the broth and cornstarch until dissolved. Add it and the tomatoes to the skillet.
6. Lower the temperature to med-low. Simmer for about two minutes.

Yields: Four servings

Cal: 177.8 | P: 18.7 g | C: 22.1 g | F: 1.8 g

Chicken Creole

Ingredients

4 chicken breasts – 1-inch strips – skinless and boneless

1 cup low-sodium chili sauce

1 can (14 ounces) cut up tomatoes

¼ cup onion

½ cup celery

1 ½ cups green peppers (1 large)

2 minced garlic cloves

1 tablespoon fresh

- Basil
- Parsley

¼ teaspoon each:

- Crushed red pepper
- Salt

Instructions

1. Chop the veggies.
2. Lightly grease a pan with some cooking spray.
3. Warm the pan on the high setting. Cook the chicken for three to five minutes.
4. Lower the temperature and blend in the remainder of the fixings.

5. Once it starts to boil, cover and simmer for ten minutes.
6. Serve over a bed of rice (calories not included in counts).

Yields: One serving

Cal: 269.3| P: 32.8 g | C: 20.7 g | F: 6.3 g

Chicken Enchiladas and Sour Cream

Ingredients

½ can (14.5 ounces) each:

- Fat-free cream of chicken soup
- Mexican Rotel

1 cup fat-free sour cream

12 ounces cooked shredded chicken breast

1 tablespoon fresh chopped cilantro

½ chopped white/yellow onion

16 corn tortillas

1 cup shredded Colby/pepper jack cheese blend (reduced-fat)

Instructions

1. Mix the soup, sour cream, and cilantro in a saucepan. Heat and set to the side.
2. Grease a skillet with a small amount of oil or cooking spray. Blend the Rotel, chicken, and onions into a pan.
3. Warm the tortillas in the microwave until they are flexible.
4. Divide all of the ingredients between the tortillas and add them to the prepared dish.

5. Empty the cream sauce over the tortillas along with the rest of the cheese.
6. Bake 30 minutes at 350ºF.

Yields: Eight servings (2 enchiladas each)

Cal: 252.0 | P: 18.3 g | C: 35.0 g | F: 4.5 g

Chicken Tetrazzini

Ingredients

1 tablespoon reduced calorie margarine

8 ounces sliced button mushrooms

½ cup chopped scallions – approximately 5

3 tablespoons all-purpose flour

¼ teaspoon garlic powder

Pinch of black pepper

½ pounds chicken breasts – cooked and cubed

1 cup fat-free chicken broth

¼ cup pimentos (2-ounce jar)

½ cup fat-free skim milk

2 tablespoons sherry cooking wine

8 ounces uncooked spaghetti

3 ½ tablespoons grated parmesan cheese

Instructions

1. Break the spaghetti into thirds, cook, and drain.
2. Add the margarine, scallions, and mushrooms in a pan and cook slowly for five minutes. Mix the milk, garlic powder, flour, pepper, and broth in a small

container. Blend it in and continue cooking ten minutes or until thickened.
3. Add the chicken, sherry, and pimentos. Cook about two minutes.
4. Stir in the cheese and cooked spaghetti.

Yields: Six servings (one cup each)

Cal: 167 | P: 10 g | C: 25g | F: 3 g

Cola Chicken

Ingredients

3 chicken breasts

1 cup ketchup

1 can (12 ounces) diet cola

Garnish: Chopped green onion

Instructions

1. Place the breasts of chicken into a skillet and add the cola and ketchup.
2. Place a lid on the pan. Once it boils, lower the temperature setting, and continue cooking for 45 minutes.
3. Take off the lid and increase the temperature until the sauce thickens and begins to stick to the chicken.

Yields: Three servings

Cal: 193.8| P: 16.2g | C: 21.4 g | F: 1.9 g

Creamy Italian Chicken – Slow Cooker

Ingredients

2 pounds chicken breasts (no skin or bones)

½ cup water

1 can - cream of chicken soup

1 container (reduced-fat / 8 ounces) cream cheese

1 pouch - Italian dressing mix

3 cups - long grain rice – cooked – brown or white

Instructions

1. Arrange the breasts in the slow cooker. Combine the water and dressing mix. Dump it over the breasts of chicken. Put the top on the pot, and set the timer on high for four hours. If you prefer, choose the low setting for eight hours. Move the chicken to a plate.
2. In another dish, add the cream cheese and soup. Dump the mixture into the pot. Add all ingredients back into the cooker as you gently shred the chicken.
3. Continue cooking on low until all ingredients are heated.
4. Serve with the rice.

For Best Results: Use the lower setting, so all ingredients fully integrated.

Yields: Six servings (2/3 cup chicken with ½ cup of rice)

Cal: 385.4 | P: 41.0 g | C: 24.1 g | F: 12.5 g

Fifteen Minute Chili

Ingredients

½ cup chopped onions

1 pound ground turkey

1 can each of the beans (16 ounces):

- Pinto
- Kidney

1 can of (28 ounces) chopped stewed tomatoes

1 tablespoon each:

- Cumin powder
- Chili powder

½ cup salsa

Instructions

1. Rinse and drain the kidney and pinto beans.
2. Brown the turkey and onions in a large soup pot.
3. Empty the tomatoes, beans, cumin, salsa, chili powder, and garlic into the pot. Cook until boiling and serve.
4. Garnish with some cheese (count the carbs).

Yields: Four servings

Cal: 370.8 | P: 31.3 g | C: 32.3 g | F: 13.3 g

Greek Yogurt Chicken

Ingredients

4 (4 ounces each) chicken breasts

1 teaspoon garlic powder

1 cup plain Greek yogurt

½ teaspoon pepper

1 ½ teaspoons seasoning salt

½ cup grated parmesan cheese

Instructions

1. Debone and remove the skin from the chicken.
2. Set the oven temperature to 375ºF.
3. Foil line a baking sheet and spray with some cooking oil.
4. Mix all of the seasonings together and coat the breasts evenly before adding to the prepared pan.
5. Bake for 45 minutes.

Yields: Four servings

Cal: 266 | P: 46 g | C: 3 g | F: 4 g

Hawaiian Turkey Burgers

Ingredients

40 ounces ground turkey

1 can (20 ounces) pineapple in unsweetened juice

2 tablespoons each:

- Minced garlic
- Ketchup

1 tablespoon each:

- Black pepper
- White vinegar

¼ teaspoon each:

- Red pepper flakes
- Salt

6 slices turkey bacon

Instructions

1. Dice the bacon into small bits and cook in a pan. Set aside in a dish. Drain and reserve the juice from the pineapple.
2. Mix the turkey, ¾ cup of the crushed pineapple, pepper, and salt in a large mixing dish.
3. In another dish, combine the ketchup, pepper flakes, pineapple juice, vinegar, and soy sauce.

4. Form the patties into 24 portions and arrange (not touching) in a baking dish. You may need two pans. Pour the pineapple juice mixture over the patties and refrigerate, covered for about an hour, turning after 30 minutes.
5. Cook the patties on a George Forman grill for two minutes or one minute on each side on a regular grill.

Yields: 24 servings

Cal: 92 | P: 9.4 g | C: 3.1 g | F: 4.1 g

Peanut Applesauce Chicken

Ingredients

1 jar (15 ounces) unsweetened applesauce

2.5 pounds - chicken pieces

½ cup powdered peanuts

¼ cup yellow mustard

1/8 cup unpacked Splenda brown sugar

To Taste: Pepper and salt

Instructions

1. Prepare the chicken in a sauté pan. When it is almost done (five minutes or so), add the powdered peanuts, sugar, mustard, and applesauce.
2. Stir and simmer over the medium heat setting on the stovetop. The internal temperature should reach 165ºF.

Yields: Eight servings

Cal: 50 | P: 3 g | C: 13 g | F: 2 g

Ranch Cheddar Turkey Burgers

Ingredients

¼ cup chopped scallion

1 pound lean ground turkey

1 (one ounce) pouch dry ranch dressing mix

1 cup low-fat shredded cheese

Instructions

1. Mix all of the fixings and form six patties.
2. Cook on the grill/skillet about six to seven minutes for each side.
3. Enjoy with tomato and lettuce on a bun (not included in counts).

Yields: Six servings

Cal: 155.1 | P: 19.3 g | C: 3.6 g | F: 6.7 g

Turkey Bean Enchilada

Ingredients

2 cups white turkey meat

6 medium scallions

1 cup taco/enchilada sauce – divided

1 can of (15 ounces) pinto beans

4 tortillas – medium sized

½ cup reduced-fat shredded Mexican cheese

Instructions

1. Cook and discard any bones or fat from the turkey while cutting it into cubes.
2. Chop the green and white parts of the scallions. Drain and rinse the pinto beans.
3. Program the oven temperature in advance to 350ºF.
4. Mix the beans, turkey, scallions, and ½ of the chosen sauce.
5. Fill each of the four tortillas, fold in the sides, and top/bottom.
6. Seam side down; add them to a casserole dish. Empty the remainder of the sauce on top of the enchiladas and cover with the cheese.
7. Place foil over the pan and bake about 20 minutes.

Yields: Four servings

Cal: 175 | P: 14 g | C: 19 g | F: 3 g

Thai Noodle Salad

Ingredients

6 ounces dried vermicelli

1 ½ cups shredded/chopped - cooked chicken

¼ cup each of low-sodium:

- Vegetable broth
- Soy sauce

½ teaspoon - crushed red peppers

2 tablespoons peanut butter

1 teaspoon each freshly minced:

- Garlic
- Ginger

1 tablespoon fresh lime juice

3 green onions

1 sweet red pepper

Lime wedges - garnish

Instructions

1. Slice the peppers into thin strips, and diagonally slice the onions into ½-inch pieces.
2. Prepare the noodles and drain.

3. Mix in a medium saucepan: the broth, soy sauce, peanut butter, red pepper, ginger, and lime juice.
4. Blend in the pasta and toss. Add the chicken, red peppers, cilantro, and onions.
5. Garnish with the lime wedges and serve to get 100% of your daily vitamin C.

Yields: Four servings

Cal: 235.9| P: 19.4 g | C: 26 g | F: 6.6 g

Chapter 2: Seafood

Breaded Cod Fillet

Ingredients

4 (6 ounces) skinless cod

Non-stick cooking spray

¼ teaspoon black pepper

¾ teaspoon fine sea salt

3 tablespoons –divided-unsalted melted margarine

¼ cup dried whole wheat bread crumbs

Juice of 1 lemon – divided

2 tablespoons chopped chives

3 tablespoons finely chopped parsley

Instructions

1. Program the oven to 425ºF.
2. Lightly coat a casserole dish with the cooking spray.
3. Flavor the cod with the pepper and salt and place in the dish.

4. Drizzle half of the lemon juice and margarine over the fish.
5. Mix the chives, parsley, and breadcrumbs in a bowl. Sprinkle it over the cod along with the remainder of lemon and margarine.
6. Bake for approximately 12 minutes.

Yields: Four servings (six ounces each)

Cal: 150 | P: 11 g | C: 6 g | F: 9 g

Crab Melt Sandwich

Ingredients

2 hard-boiled, chopped egg whites

12 ounces imitation crabmeat (coarsely chopped)

2 tablespoons chopped onion

4 tablespoons light mayonnaise

Dash of black pepper

¼ cup shredded Swiss cheese

4 slices of each:

- ¼-inch tomatoes
- Whole-wheat bread

Instructions

1. Mix the crab, egg whites, and onion, pepper, and mayonnaise.
2. Arrange the sliced of bread on the broiler pan topping with the tomatoes, crab, and mayo mixture.
3. Sprinkle each one with the Swiss cheese and broil.
- **Note**: You can use real crab but would need to adjust the counts.

Yields: Four servings

Cal: 296.3 | P: 20.3 g | C: 32.4 g | F: 9.6 g

Mock Crab Cakes

Ingredients

2 egg whites

2 pounds imitation crabmeat

1 sleeve (34) Keebler Toasteds/or other crackers – crushed

4 tablespoons light mayonnaise

Instructions

1. Program the temperature in the oven to 375ºF.
2. Whisk the eggs until fluffy and blend in the mayonnaise
3. Add the crushed crackers with the eggs and combine with the crabmeat.
4. Make the patties using about ½- cup for each patty.
5. Bake 15 minutes per side.

Yields: 10 servings

Cal: 161.4 | P: 7.4 g | C: 21.6 g | F: 4.4 g

Rainbow Trout – Pan-Fried

Ingredients

8 ounces rainbow trout fillets

1 1/3 tablespoons chopped parsley

3 tablespoons yellow cornmeal

¼ teaspoon each:

- Black pepper
- Ground celery seeds

2 teaspoons olive oil

1 pinch salt

Instructions

1. Clean and rinse the fillets in cold water. Pat them dry.
2. Blend the pepper, cornmeal, salt, parsley, and celery to coat the fish.
3. Warm the oil in a frying pan and cook each side for two to three minutes.
4. Enjoy when they are easily flaked with a fork.

Yields: Six servings

Cal: 240 | P: 25 g | C: 10 g | F: 10 g

Salmon

BBQ Roasted Salmon

Ingredients

4 (6 ounces) salmon fillets

2 tbsp. fresh lemon juice

¼ cup pineapple juice

2 tbsp. brown sugar

½ tsp. salt

2 tsp. grated lemon rind

¾ tsp. ground cumin

4 tsp. chili powder

¼ tsp. cinnamon

Instructions

1. Program the oven temperature to 400ºF.
2. Add the first three ingredients into a Ziploc plastic bag. Marinate for a minimum of one hour—turning occasionally.

3. Remove the salmon and throw the marinade in the trash.
4. Combine the rest of the ingredients and rub it over the fish.
5. Arrange them in a lightly coated baking dish for 12 to 15 minutes.
6. Garnish with some lemon.

Yields: Four servings

Cal: 225 | P: 34 g | C: 7 g | F: 6 g

Mediterranean Salmon with Pasta

Ingredients

4 (4 ounces) salmon fillets (16 ounces total)

2 medium sliced tomatoes

1 medium red bell pepper

4 cups whole wheat spaghetti - cooked

To Taste:

- Black pepper
- Lemon juice

2 tablespoons prepared pesto

Garnish: Drizzle of olive oil

Instructions

1. Slice the peppers into thin slices.
2. Program the oven setting to 400ºF.
3. Arrange each of the fillets on the center of aluminum foil along with a ½ tablespoon each of the pesto sauce. Divide the veggies on/around the fish. Sprinkle with pepper and enclose the foil.
4. Bake 15 to 20 minutes.

Yields: Four servings

Cal: 407.5 | P: 38.7 g | C: 44.9 g | F: 9.2 g

Quick and Easy Salmon

Ingredients

12 ounces fresh salmon

¼ cup each soy sauce

Maple syrup/honey (not pancake syrup)

2-3 minced garlic cloves

Instructions

1. Combine all of the fixings into a Ziploc bag and shake. Place the salmon in the bag of fixings, and let it rest for a minimum of one hour in the refrigerator.
2. Mix all of the components into a baking dish and cover with a layer of aluminum foil.
3. Bake for fifteen minutes in a preheated oven at 350ºF.

Yields: Four servings (3 ounces each)

Cal: 183.1 | P: 18.0 g | C: 14.9 g | F: 5.5 g

Salmon Patties

Ingredients

¼ cup green bell pepper

½ of a medium onion

1 stalk of celery

1 can of pink salmon

½ cup breadcrumbs

1 egg

½ teaspoon each:

- Chili powder
- **Optional**: Old Bay Seasoning

Instructions

1. Chop the pepper, onion, and celery into fine bits.
2. Clean the salmon by discarding the bones and skin.
3. Mix the egg, veggies, breadcrumbs, salmon, and seasonings together.
4. Scoop them out and add to a well-greased griddle.
5. Smash the patty and cook five minutes per side.
6. Top with a bit of ketchup or horseradish.

Yields: Four servings

Cal: 216.8 | P: 26 g | C: 11 g | F: 8 g

Shrimp

Creole Shrimp

Ingredients

2 teaspoons canola oil

1 chopped onion - 1 ½ cups

2 each chopped:

- Bell peppers
- Garlic cloves

3 chopped celery stalks

½ teaspoon:

- Paprika
- Thyme

¼ teaspoon:

- Cayenne pepper
- Black pepper

2 cups of each:

- Brown cooked rice
- Vegetable stock

1 cup tomato sauce – no salt added

2 tablespoons tomato paste

12 ounces peeled – deveined shrimp

Instructions

1. Using medium heat, saute the onions for two minutes. Toss in the celery and garlic and saute two more minutes; lastly, the tomato paste, spices and peppers cooking another two minutes.
2. Add the tomato sauce and stock into the pan another two minutes stirring to a boil.
3. Simmer about ten minutes and add the shrimp. Simmer two minutes.
4. Serve over rice.

Yields: 1 ¼ cup servings of Creole and ½ cup rice (four servings total)

Cal: 302.1 | P: 22.8 g | C: 45.1 g | F: 4.9 g

–

Lime Shrimp

Ingredients

28 large ready to cook shrimp

2 dashes salt

½ lime – juiced

2 tablespoons chopped onion

¾ teaspoon black pepper

Instructions

1. Toss all of the components into a skillet on medium heat. Toss and enjoy!

Yields: Two servings

Cal: 84.4 | P: 16.3 g | C: 2.2 g | F: 0.9 g

Shrimp Pasta

Ingredients

1 pound fresh medium shrimp

8 ounces each:

- Fettuccine
- Cream cheese (reduced-fat)

1 cup of each:

- Chicken broth
- Grated parmesan cheese

2 garlic cloves

5 ounces frozen spinach – thawed – moisture removed

To Taste: Pepper and salt

Instructions

1. Prepare the fettuccine.
2. Heat a skillet using the med-high setting. Add the chicken broth and cream cheese, stirring three to four minutes until it's well blended.
3. Add the garlic, pepper, and salt, along with the parmesan cheese.
4. Stir in the shrimp and stir until completely done. Toss in the spinach. Stir and enjoy.

Yields: Six servings

Cal: 363.5| P: 30.9g | C: 24.0 g | F: 15.2 g

Tilapia

Broiled Tilapia Parmesan

Ingredients

1 pound tilapia fillets

1 tbsp. (+) 1 ½ tsp. reduced fat mayonnaise

2 tbsp. softened butter

1/8 tsp. each of:

- Onion powder
- Ground black pepper
- Dried basil
- Celery seed

1 tbsp. fresh lemon juice

Instructions

1. Preheat the broiler on the oven. Line with foil or grease a broiling pan.
2. Combine the butter, mayonnaise, parmesan cheese, and lemon juice in a small container. Toss in the onion powder, pepper, basil, and celery salt. Stir and set to the side.

3. Place the fillets into the baking pan and broil two to three minutes. Flip them once and broil two more minutes.
4. Take the fish from the oven and coat them with the cheese mixture. Broil two more minutes.

Yields: Four servings

Cal: 177.1 | P: 19.6 g | C: 1.2 g | F: 10.5g

Lemon Garlic Tilapia

Ingredients

1 tablespoon each:

- Butter/margarine
- Olive oil

4 tilapia fillets

Juice of 1 lemon

Dash of salt

To Taste: Cayenne pepper

1 teaspoon each:

- Parsley flakes
- Garlic salt

Instructions

1. Program the oven to 400ºF.
2. Place the butter in a microwavable dish along with the salt, oil, juice, parsley, and garlic powder. Saute a few minutes. Pour it over the fillets in a baking pan.
3. Sprinkle the top of the fish with the cayenne. Bake 13 minutes, and broil for another two to three minutes.

Yields: Four servings

Cal: 175.2 | P: 26.1 g | C: 1.8 g | F: 7.3 g

Oven-Fried Tilapia

Ingredients

3 egg whites

One pound (4) tilapia fillets

1 tablespoon each:

- Onion powder
- Garlic powder
- Grated parmesan cheese
- Cajun seasoning

1 ½ cups finely ground Fiber One cereal/oven-fry bread

Non-stick cooking spray

Instructions

1. Program the oven temperature to 400ºF.
2. Whisk the egg whites until frothy.
3. In a separate container, combine all of the seasonings, cheese, and cereal.
4. Lightly spray a cookie sheet and add the fish. Spritz a small amount of oil directly on the fish.
5. Bake 8 to 10 minutes.

Yields: Four servings (4 ounces each)

Cal: 184.7 | P: 27.9 g | C: 22.1 g | F: 3.1 g

Tuna

Best Ever Tuna Salad

Ingredients

2/3 cup cottage cheese (non-fat)

1 can of albacore tuna

4 tablespoons plain low-fat yogurt

1 stalk of celery

¼ small onion

1 teaspoon Dijon mustard

Pinch of dill

Splash lemon juice

Instructions

1. Finely chop the onion and celery.
2. Get a big dish for two and have lunch with all of the goodies in a bowl. (Of course, make them even servings.)

Yields: Two servings

Cal: 190.3 | P: 32.5 g | C: 11.7 g | F: 2.2 g

Crunchy Tuna Patties

Ingredients

4 egg whites

4 cans (3 ounces) tuna packed in water

¼ cup each:

- Chopped water chestnuts/diced red pepper/capers
- Grated carrot

16 crushed Wheat Thin crackers

1 tablespoon minced onion

To Taste

- Dried mustard
- Dill
- Pepper

Instructions

1. Combine all of the fixings and form eight patties.
2. Use cooking oil to spray a skillet. Over medium temperature on the stovetop, brown the patties two to three minutes for each side.

Yields: Eight servings

Cal: 80 | P: 12 g | C: 4 g | F: 1 g

Tuna and White Bean Salad

Ingredients

1 can of (15.5 ounces) chickpeas/white beans

2 cans tuna (chunk light in water)

1 red bell pepper

¼ cup onion

Juice of 1 lemon

1 tablespoon olive oil

Optional

- Spinach
- Tomatoes
- Parsley

Instructions

1. Drain and rinse the beans. Drain the tuna. Dice the onion and pepper.
2. Combine all of the goodies and chill for a minimum of four hours.

3. Serve over a bed of greens.

Yields: Four servings

Cal: 193.2 | P: 22.6 g | C: 20.4 | F: 4.3 g

Chapter 3: Soups

Barley and Beef Soup

Ingredients

1 pound beef – stew meat/chuck/steak

1 tablespoon butter

½ cup each chopped:

- Carrots
- Onions
- Celery

4 cups each:

- Water
- Beef broth

¾ cup barley (quick-cook)

1 teaspoon each:

- Salt
- Black pepper

½ teaspoon each:

- Oregano
- Basil

1 can of (14.5 ounces) diced tomatoes

Instructions

1. Put the butter in a soup kettle and saute the celery, carrot, and onion for about five minutes.
2. Pour in the water, broth, tomatoes, beef, pepper, salt, barley, basil, and oregano. When it begins to boil, lower the temperature and cook about twenty minutes to an hour depending on how you like its consistency.

Yields: 12servings

Cal: 198.6 | P: 13.7 g | C: 16.3 g | F: 8.7 g

Cabbage Vegetable Soup

Ingredients

1 medium diced onion

1 can each:

- 28 ounces - crushed tomatoes
- 14.5 ounces green beans
- 15 ounces can pinto beans
- 12 ounces sweet yellow corn

3 medium diced carrots

1 head shredded cabbage

3 diced stalks of celery

Instructions

1. Pour the tomatoes, cabbage, celery, onion, and carrots in a pot. Simmer about 20 minutes over medium heat.
2. Add the canned veggies and serve.

Yields: Six servings (1 ½ cups each)

Cal: 165.2 | P: 8.3 g | C: 36.6 g | F: 1.8 g

Chicken Taco Stew – Slow Cooker

Ingredients

2 chicken breasts – no bones or skin

2 cans diced tomatoes w/chilies (14 ½ oz. each)

1 chopped onion

1 can tomato sauce (8 oz.)

1 can corn (16 oz.)

1 can each of 16 oz. beans:

- Kidney
- Black

1 package of taco seasoning (1.25 ounces)

Instructions

1. Mix all of the fixings except for the chicken in the crock pot.
2. Arrange the breasts on top and cover with the lid.
3. Cook on the high setting for three to four hours. If you prefer, you can choose the low setting for six to eight hours.
4. Shred the chicken about 30 minutes before you are ready to serve.
5. Blend it back into the soup pot and heat until you are ready to eat.

Yields: 14 servings – 1 cup each

Cal: 158.7| P: 14 g | C: 24.4 g | F: 1.1 g

Chicken Tortilla Soup – Slow Cooker

Ingredients

1 lb. frozen chicken

1 medium chopped onion

1 can of:

- Whole peeled tomatoes (15 oz.)
- Enchilada sauce (10 oz.)
- Chopped green chile peppers (4 oz.)
- Black beans – rinsed (15 oz.)

3 cans (14.5 oz. each) chicken broth

1 pkg. frozen corn (10 oz.)

1 teaspoon cumin

2 minced garlic cloves

¼ teaspoon black pepper

Instructions

1. Arrange the chicken, enchilada sauce, tomatoes, green chiles, onions, and garlic into the crock pot.
2. Flavor the pot fixings with the pepper, salt, and cumin. Empty the chicken broth, black beans, and corn. Cook low for six to eight hrs. or high for three hrs.

186

3. Garnish with some shredded cheese, avocados, sour cream or other ingredients of your choosing. Be sure to add the additional calories.

Yields: Eight servings

Cal: 169.1 | P: 17.4 g | C: 20.3 g | F: 2.5 g

Corn Chowder Soup

Ingredients

1 tablespoon olive oil

1 package frozen whole kernel corn (10 ounces)

2 tbsp. each finely diced:

- Green pepper
- Onion
- Celery
- Chopped fresh parsley

1 cup each of:

- Peeled – diced potatoes
- Water

Pepper if desired

¼ teaspoon each:

- Salt
- Paprika

2 cups low-fat/skim milk

¼ cup minced fresh parsley

2 tablespoons flour

Instructions

1. Pour the oil into a skillet on the stovetop using the medium heat setting. Also, add the celery, onion,

and green peppers into a pan and saute for two minutes.
2. Blend in the potatoes, corn, pepper, salt, water, and paprika. Let it boil and lower the temperature to the medium setting and continue cooking for ten minutes.
3. Mix the flour in a jar with a ½ cup of milk, and shake. Blend it in with the cooked veggies along with the rest of the milk.
4. Cook until it thickens and garnish with parsley.

Yields: Four – 1 cup servings

Cal: 202.5 | P: 8.0 g | C: 32.7 g | F: 5.3 g

Curried Carrot Soup

Ingredients

½ pound chopped carrots

½ tbsp. of olive oil (extra-virgin)

1 garlic clove

1 tsp. curry powder

¼-inch piece fresh mashed ginger

3 cups vegetable broth – low sodium

¼ cup light coconut milk

Instructions

1. Add the oil to a skillet on the stovetop using the high heat setting. Toss in the garlic, ginger, curry powder, carrots, and 1 ½ cups of the vegetable broth.
2. When it begins to boil, reduce the temperature, and cook until the carrots are soft (15 to 20 minutes). Pour in the remainder of the vegetable broth.
3. Puree the mixture in the blender when they are mushy and have cooled.
4. Add the puree back into the pot and heat on medium high, pouring in the milk.
5. Serve warm and enjoy with a sprinkle of freshly cracked black pepper.

Yields: Four servings

Cal: 63.4 | P: 0.7 g | C: 8.4 g | F: 2.9 g